EPIDEMIOLOGY
AND
BIOSTATISTICS

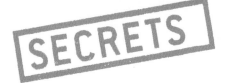

EPIDEMIOLOGY AND BIOSTATISTICS

SECRETS

Robert J. Nordness, MD, MPH
Formerly, Officer in Charge
Naval Undersea Medical Institute
Groton, Connecticut

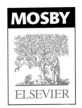

MOSBY

ELSEVIER

1600 John F. Kennedy Boulevard, Suite 1800
Philadelphia, PA 19103-2899

Epidemiology and Biostatistics Secrets

ISBN-13: 978-0-323-03406-7
ISBN-10: 0-323-03406-3

Copyright © 2006, Elsevier Inc. All rights reserved.

NOTICE

ISBN-13: 978-0-323-03406-7
ISBN-10: 0-323-03406-3

Vice President, Medical Education: Linda Belfus
Developmental Editor: Stan Ward
Senior Project Manager: Cecelia Bayruns
Marketing Manager: Kate Rubin

Printed in China.

Last digit is the print number: 9   8   7   6   5   4   3

CONTENTS

I. EPIDEMIOLOGY

II. BIOSTATISTICS

CONTRIBUTORS

Robbie Ali, MD, MPH, MPPM
Visiting Associate Professor, Department of Behavioral and Community Health Sciences, University of Pittsburgh Graduate School of Public Health, Pittsburgh, Pennsylvania

Adam M. Brown, DO
Instructor, Naval Undersea Medical Institute, Groton, Connecticut

Mark Glover, BA, BM, BCh, MRCGP, MFOM
Consultant Occupant Physician, Undersea Medicine Division, Institute of Naval Medicine, Alverstoke, Gosport, Hampshire, United Kingdom

Moore H. Jan, MD, MPH
Head, Occupational Medicine, U.S. Naval Medical Center and Branch Clinics, Portsmouth, Virginia

Christopher Jankosky, MD, MPH
Chief Resident, Department of Occupational Medicine, Johns Hopkins School of Public Health, Baltimore, Maryland

John L. Kane, MD
Great Lakes Naval Hospital, Great Lakes, Illinois

Sue Kim, MD
Division of Hematology, Stanford University Medical Center, Stanford, California

Michael D. Lappi, DO, PhD
Department of Occupational and Environmental Medicine, Harvard Medical School, Boston, Massachusetts

Patrick R. Laraby, MD, MBA, MPH, FACOEM
Head, Occupational and Environmental Health, Naval Hospital, Naples, Italy

Jonathan M. Lieske, MD, MPH
Senior Medical Officer, Naval Special Warfare Group Two, Norfolk, Virginia

Neal Andrew Naito, MD, MPH
Head, Occupational Health Clinic, National Naval Medical Center; Adjunct Assistant Research Professor, Uniformed Services University of the Health Sciences, Bethesda, Maryland

Mark Nordness, MD
ProHealth Care, Inc., Waukesha, Wisconsin

Robert J. Nordness, MD, MPH
Formerly, Officer in Charge, Naval Undersea Medical Institute, Groton, Connecticut

Lee Okurowski, MD, MPH, MBA
South Walpole, Massachusetts

Philip D. Parks, MD, MPH
Diving Medical Officer, Naval Special Warfare Group Two, United States Navy, Norfolk, Virginia

Robert W. Perkins, MD, MPH
Medical Corps, United States Navy, Poulsbo, Washington

Ward L. Reed, MD, MPH
Naval Aerospace Medicine Institute, Pensacola, Florida

Ashita Tolwani, MD, MSc
Division of Nephrology, Department of Medicine, University of Alabama at Birmingham School of Medicine, Birmingham, Alabama

Thomas H. Winters, MD, FACOEM, FACPM
President and Chief Medical Officer, Occupational and Environmental Health Network; Lecturer, Harvard School of Public Health and Harvard Medical School, Boston, Massachusetts

Richard I. Wittman, MD, MPH
Associate Medical Director, Workforce Medical Center, Redwood City, California

Ann M. Zaia, NP-C, SM, MSN, MHA, CHS-III, CHE, COHN-S
Sudbury, Massachusetts

PREFACE

The art of clinical decision-making rests on a foundation composed of knowledge and experience in the medical field. Never in history have clinicians been inundated with such a barrage of published information meant to be useful in the care of patients, yet many accomplished caregivers feel their ability to use the current medical literature effectively is lacking. This book is meant to serve as both a primer and a refresher for some of the fundamental concepts in epidemiology and biostatistics for health care workers of all levels of experience. A more comprehensive, focused, and/or theoretical perspective on any of the topics introduced can be obtained within the rich variety of texts available in the fields of epidemiology and biostatistics.

Robert J. Nordness, MD, MPH

DEDICATION

To my children

Daniel, Oscar, and Claire

who are my life.

TOP 100 SECRETS

These secrets are 100 of the top board alerts. They summarize the concepts, principles, and most salient details of epidemiology and biostatistics.

1. Epidemiology is the study of the distribution and determinants of disease in the human population. It is the basic science and fundamental practice of public health.

2. Some underlying premises of epidemiology are that human disease does not occur at random, and that causal and preventive factors for disease can be identified through systematic investigation of different populations or population subgroups in varying places or times.

3. Descriptive epidemiology is concerned with identifying the general characteristics of the distribution of disease, particularly in relation to person, place, and time. Descriptive studies include ecologic (i.e., correlation) studies, case reports and case series, and cross-section surveys.

4. Analytic epidemiology requires a study to test a specific hypothesis regarding the relationship between an exposure to a risk factor and an outcome, typically a disease. Both observational and experimental studies are considered analytic studies, but only in experimental studies is the exposure determined by the researcher.

5. Generally, crude rates of morbidity or mortality must be adjusted to be useful in comparing different populations. Adjusted rates are also termed *standardized rates,* with age distribution being the most common adjusted factor.

6. The following three levels of prevention are considered in public health:
   - Primary prevention: the prevention of disease or injury (e.g., health promotions programs and immunizations)
   - Secondary prevention: the early detection and prompt treatment of disease (e.g., screening programs)
   - Tertiary prevention: the reduction of disability and the promotion of rehabilitation from disease (e.g., surgical corrections and rehabilitation programs)

7. Risk factors for disease—or health—can be genetic, environmental, or lifestyle-related. The combination of these factors can profoundly affect risk for a given individual. Whenever possible, interpret risk in terms of actual numbers of events, taking into account background risk and the prevalence of exposure to risk factors.

8. A rate has a denominator with units that include time (e.g., 25 deaths per 100,000 population per year). A risk does not require time within the denominator (e.g., 2.6 deaths per 100 open-heart operations). Always check the denominator in a risk calculation to establish exactly what population provides the source of the observations.

9. A relative risk (RR), or risk ratio, is a measure of the absolute risk in one population as a proportion of the absolute risk in another. Usually, but not invariably, the higher risk is used for the numerator.

10. The odds ratio can be calculated for both cohort and case-control studies, although relative risk cannot be calculated for a case-control study. When the outcome is rare, however, the odds ratio is a good approximation for relative risk.

11. Attributable risk, defined as the additional risk of disease in an exposed group over that in an unexposed group, is influenced by the magnitude of background risk, whereas relative risk is not.

12. The incidence rate is the number of new cases of a disease in a specified period divided by the population at risk during that period. Prevalence is the number of people with a disease at a given point or period divided by the population at risk at that given point or period. Prevalence can be estimated by multiplying the incidence rate by the average duration of the condition.

13. As data-gathering instruments, surveys are cross-sectional, meaning that information regarding both exposure and outcome are collected simultaneously. In cross-section surveys it is impossible to ascertain any information about the temporal relationship between a potential risk factor and its outcome. Surveys are useful in identifying those with chronic or less severe disease processes because subjects are more likely to be present and healthy enough to participate, as opposed to subjects suffering from severe, rapidly progressive diseases.

14. Surveillance is the systematic collection, analysis, and dissemination of disease data about groups of people, and is designed to detect early signs of disease. Surveillance is performed at many levels for a large variety of populations and is a cornerstone of preventive medicine. Its primary purpose is to prevent disease and injury and, ultimately, to improve quality of life.

15. Baseline rates set the standard by which all future occurrences of an event (e.g., sick days or cancer) may be compared to detect atypical patterns, such as an epidemic.

16. The National Center for Health Statistics (NCHS) collects vital statistics in the United States. Vital Statistics are critical events in the life span of an individual; in the United States, these events are birth, death, marriage, divorce, and fetal death.

17. The Bureau of Labor Statistics is the principal fact-finding agency for the federal government for topics relating to labor economics and statistics, such as inflation, wages, productivity, health, demographics, and unemployment.

18. The epidemiologic triangle is comprised of a host, an agent, and an environment. A host is a living organism capable of becoming infected, an agent is a factor that must be present (or potentially missing) for the occurrence of a disease, and an environment is an extrinsic force or situation affecting the host's opportunity to be exposed to an agent.

19. *Direct transmission* is the transfer of an infectious agent by physical contact with lesions, blood, saliva, or other secretion; *indirect transmission* occurs when the infectious agent spends a variable period within or upon some intermediary substance or living organism.

20. Infectivity is the proportion of persons who, exposed to a causative agent, eventually develop an infectious disease. Pathogenicity is the ability of an organism to cause a diseased state (i.e., morbidity). Virulence is the ability to cause death (i.e., mortality).

21. An epidemic, or outbreak, is simply a higher frequency of disease or injury than is expected for a typical population and time period.

22. The 10 steps of an outbreak investigation are as follows:
    - Prepare for field work.
    - Establish the existence of an outbreak.

- Verify the diagnosis.
- Define and identify cases.
- Describe and orient the data in terms of time, place, and person.
- Develop hypotheses.
- Evaluate hypotheses.
- Refine hypotheses and carry out additional studies.
- Implement control and prevention measures.
- Communicate findings.

23. An association can be due to the following four mechanisms:
    - Spuriousness (i.e., artifactual): the association results from error or bias in the study design, implementation, or analysis.
    - Confounding: the relationship between an exposure and the development of a disease is distorted by an additional variable.
    - Chance: an observed association is due to chance alone.
    - Causation: a factor directly or indirectly causes an observed outcome.

24. The Hill Criteria for causality are as follows:
    - Strength of the association
    - Consistency
    - Specificity
    - Temporality
    - Biologic gradient
    - Plausibility
    - Coherence
    - Experimental evidence
    - Analogy

25. There are four types of causal relations:
    - Necessary and sufficient
    - Necessary but not sufficient
    - Sufficient but not necessary
    - Neither sufficient nor necessary

26. Confounding occurs when an exposure-outcome association occurs solely because a distinct third factor is associated with both exposure and outcome. The observed association is true but not causal.

27. Effect modification occurs when the effect of a risk factor on a particular outcome varies with the presence and/or level of a third variable. This third variable is called an *effect modifier* because it modifies the effect (i.e., outcome) of the risk factor.

28. The "healthy worker effect" describes the phenomenon that workers as a group are usually healthier than the unemployed. Not only are the healthy more likely to obtain employment, but also, once employed, are more likely to have employer-based insurance, which improves their access to health care.

29. Bias is a systematic error in the design, implementation, and/or analysis of a study, causing a false estimate, which usually skews observations in one direction. The two major classifications of bias are selection and observation (i.e., information).

30. Descriptive studies include the following:
    - Correlation studies (e.g., studies of populations or ecologic studies)
    - Case reports
    - Case series
    - Cross-section surveys

31. Analytic studies include the following:
    - Observational studies (e.g., case-control studies or cohort studies)
    - Intervention studies (e.g., clinical trials)

32. In a case-control study, subjects who develop a condition (i.e., cases) and subjects who have not developed a condition (i.e., controls) are selected, and the two groups are compared with respect to prior exposure.

33. In a cohort study, subjects are defined by the presence or absence of an exposure to a suspected risk factor for a disease; these subjects are then studied over time. The relative frequency of the outcome of interest is analyzed to determine whether the exposure is indeed a risk factor for the disease.

34. The intervention trial model compares different treatment protocols or preventive interventions provided to various groups of subjects, with the outcome compared between the groups. The randomized controlled trial (RCT) is a type of intervention model that provides the strongest evidence regarding the relationship between intervention and outcome.

35. When using a medical article to answer clinical questions, always ask the following questions:
    - Are the results of the study valid?
    - Is the evidence important?
    - How can the valid and important results be applied to patient care?

36. The following is the hierarchy of evidence used in evidence-based medicine, listed from most to least useful:
    - N of 1 randomized controlled trials
    - A systematic review of randomized controlled trials
    - A single randomized trial
    - A systematic review of observation studies
    - A single observation study
    - A physiologic study
    - An unsystematic clinical observation

37. Diagnostic tests with very high sensitivity values are useful for ruling out a given disease or condition when the results are negative. This can be remembered by the mnemonic **SnNout**: a **s**e**n**sitive test with a **n**egative result rules **out** a disease.

38. Diagnostic tests with very high specificity values are useful for ruling in a given disease or condition when the results are positive. This can be remembered by the mnemonic **SpPin**: a **sp**ecific test with a **p**ositive result rules **in** a disease.

39. The number needed to treat (NNT) is a numeric expression of the number of patients receiving an active treatment needed to demonstrate a benefit over no treatment. NNT is the inverse of the absolute risk reduction (ARR) and is given by the expression NNT=1/ARR.

40. Likelihood ratios measure how much a diagnostic test will raise or lower the pretest probability for a given disease or disorder. The greater the likelihood ratio positive (i.e., the ratio of sensitivity to false-positive rate), the greater the increase will be between the pretest and posttest probability.

41. Through the application of statistic principles to the biologic sciences, biostatisticians can distinguish methodically between true differences among observations and random chance variations, allowing them to determine associations between risk factors and disease to reduce illness and injury.

42. The empirical rule states that, in a normal distribution, roughly 68% of the data will be within one standard deviation (SD) of the mean, near 95% of the distribution will be within two SDs of the mean, and approximately 99.7% of the data will be within three SDs of the mean.

43. The mean, median, and mode are measures of central tendency. The median is less affected than the mean by outliers, making the median a more robust measure of central tendency and, therefore, a better measure of central tendency for skewed data.

44. The range, standard deviation, and variance are typical measures of the dispersion, or spread, of the data set being examined.

45. Sensitivity = $\dfrac{TP}{TP+FN}$ = true-positive rate = 1 − false-negative rate

46. Specificity = $\dfrac{TN}{TN+FP}$ = true-negative rate = 1 − false-positive rate

47. An asymmetric data distribution is skewed to the left (or negatively skewed) if the longer tail of the curve extends to the left; if the opposite is true, then the distribution is skewed to the right, or positively skewed. The mode is situated on the highest point on the curve, the mean is located toward the longer tail, and the median is situated between the mode and the mean.

48. A variable is anything that can be measured and is observed to fluctuate. Quantitative variables are measured on a numeric scale, while qualitative variables are measured with no natural sense of order.

49. The four typical measurement scales are as follows:
   - Nominal scales: used to arbitrarily group qualitative data
   - Ordinal scales: show rank, but give no information about the distance between values
   - Interval scales: have meaningful ranks and spacing between values
   - Ratio scales: have meaningful zeros, ranks, and spacing, all of which give meaning to the ratio of two values

50. The following are the measures central tendency:
   - Mean: the arithmetic average of the observed values, strongly affected by extreme values
   - Median: division of the distribution into two equal groups
   - Mode: the most common observed value in the distribution; there can be multiple modes within a data set

51. The following are measures of dispersion in a sample data set:
   - Range: the difference between the lowest and highest value, giving width of the distribution but nothing else
   - Standard deviation: the most commonly used measure of dispersion, calculated using the formula:

$$SD = \sqrt{\dfrac{\sum(x-\bar{x})^2}{n-1}}$$

   where S = summation of, x = individual score, $\bar{x}$ = mean of all scores, and n = sample size, or the number of scores
   - Variance: the square of standard deviation

52. Random measurement error increases dispersion, is unpredictable, and is likely to fall on either side of the true value of the property being measured. Precision is lack of random error, leading to a tight grouping with repeated measurements.

53. Systematic error (i.e., bias) causes repeated measurements to fall consistently around a value other than the true value of the property being measured. Validity is the lack of systematic error.

54. A frequency distribution illustrates how often different data categories (or ranges of values) appear within a data sample. This information may be presented in many different formats, including tables, graphs, and plots. Tabular data is useful when there are large numbers of variables to display.

55. In a frequency distribution, an area under the curve bounded by limiting values is proportional to the percentage of the sample data falling between those limits.

56. The means of repeated samples from a population tend to be normally distributed, even when the population they are taken from is not. This phenomenon is described by the central limit theorem.

57. The standard error of the mean describes the dispersion of sample means about the population mean in the same way that the standard deviation describes the dispersion of sample values about the sample mean.

58. In a random sample for a dichotomous event or trait, it is improbable (but not impossible) to sample a proportion of that trait that is very different from the population purely by chance. Binomial distributions quantify that likelihood.

59. There is a different binomial distribution for every combination of sample size *(n)* and base probability *(p)*.

60. A histogram is a graphical representation of a given frequency distribution in which rectangles are drawn with their bases representing a given interval; the areas of the rectangles are proportional to the number of frequency values within the interval spanned. In histograms, information about the extremes of the distributions is often lost because of the use of the open-ended "less than" or "greater than" intervals at the extremes.

61. A frequency polygon is a graph formed by joining the midpoints of histogram column tops with straight lines. A frequency polygon smooths out abrupt changes that can occur in histogram plots and helps to demonstrate continuity.

62. A bar diagram, or bar chart, is a graphic representation of discrete data in which different categories or classifications are represented on one axis and the frequency count is represented on the other. Like histograms, the area of the bar is proportional to the count.

63. A stem-and-leaf diagram is essentially a histogram rotated on its side; stem values represent the intervals and leaves represent the frequency count in the interval. The stem in this diagram is the left-hand digits of the numeric data, whereas the leaves are the last digit to the right of the stem. The frequency, or number of leaves, of each stem value is given in a separate column.

64. A box-and-whisker plot is a visual representation of data with an arbitrarily sized box made around the value of the median, represented by a middle vertical line, with two other vertical divisions representing the first quartile (i.e., 25th percentile) and the third quartile (i.e., 75th percentile).

65. A pie diagram is a circular diagram divided into segments, each of which represents the frequency of a category. The total of the slices of the pie must add up to 100%.

66. A line graph is a useful method of displaying data over a period of time. Typically, an occurrence rate of some type is represented on the y-axis, and the time over which the occurrence is tracked is represented on the x-axis.

67. A typical null hypothesis states that there is no detected difference in outcome between two groups with different exposures. Accepting the null hypothesis means that no statistically significant difference was found in the study.

68. A type I error is, simply, declaring that a difference exists when, in fact, it does not. This error is committed by rejecting the null hypothesis when it is true. The symbol α (alpha) signifies the probability of making a type I error. A type II error is declaring that no difference exists when, in fact, a difference is present. This error is committed by accepting the null hypothesis when it is false. The symbol β (beta) signifies the probability of making a type II error.

69. Be aware that a small effect in a study with a large sample size can have the same p-value as a large effect in a small study.

70. A finding of statistical significance should not automatically lead to the conclusion of clinical importance.

71. Power is the probability of not accepting a false null hypothesis, which is equal to $1 - \beta$. Underpowered studies can probably be justified in two settings: when investigating a rare disease and when performing pilot studies on new drugs or therapies.

72. Probability quantifies the likelihood of occurrence of an event A over unlimited trials; the standard equation for estimating probability is P(event) = A/N, where N is the number of trials attempted in which A could occur.

73. The odds of an event taking place is the ratio of the probability of the event taking place to the probability of the event not taking place, as expressed by the following formula:

Odds = probability of event / (1 − probability of event)

74. The additive rule states that P(A or B) = P(A) + P(B) − P(A and B). If A and B are mutually exclusive, this equation reduces to P(A or B) = P(A) + P(B).

75. The multiplicative rule for independent events states P(A and B) = P(A) $\times$ P(B)

If two events are not independent, a special form of the multiplicative rule can be used: P(A and B) = P(A | B) P(B) = P(B | A) P(A).

76. Sampling allows a researcher to make inferences about a target population by using only a portion of the population, known as a sample. A good sample must be representative of the characteristics of the target population; randomization is a tool used to increase the probability that the sample will truly represent the parent population.

77. Estimation of sample size is performed prior to conducting a study to assess the feasibility and constraints of performing the study.

78. Predictive value is highly dependent upon the prevalence of the condition in the tested population. Positive predictive value in one test is almost always very low when the prevalence is low.

79. Always be aware that even the gold standard test has flaws.

80. Cohen's Kappa is used to give a quantitative value (from −1 to 1) regarding the degree of agreement between individual raters for a particular outcome or test, taking into account agreement due to chance.

81. The performance of a test can be altered depending on where the positive point is set. An ROC curve illustrates the effects of this variability on sensitivity and specificity.

82. Parallel testing yields a sensitive but nonspecific result; serial testing yields a specific but not sensitive result.

83. Use the *t*-test to compare a sample mean and a population mean, two independent samples, or the same sample at two different times (often before and after treatment) when the population standard deviation is unknown.

84. The *t*-distribution and normal distribution compare as follows:
    - The *t*-distribution and normal distribution are similar in three ways: both are symmetric about 0, both are bell-shaped, and both are single-peaked.
    - The *t*-distribution differs from normal distribution in that *t*-distribution has a larger tail than the normal distribution, although as the degrees of freedom increase, the distribution in the tail approaches that of a normal distribution.
    - For samples greater than 30, the *t*-distribution is nearly identical to the normal distribution (*z*-distribution).

85. A given confidence interval shows the probability that the true value of the mean lies within the stated interval.

86. Before analyzing your data, ask yourself the following questions:
    - Are your data continuous, discrete, or categorical?
    - Are the data paired?
    - Will any of the data be assumed to follow a normal distribution?
    The answers will largely determine which statistical tests or methods you can apply.

87. If you cannot or do not want to make any assumptions of normality, use a nonparametric approach. Nonparametric methods should be considered for small sample sizes.

88. A scatterplot should be the first step in the analysis of bivariate, continuous, or discrete, paired data. Pearson's correlation coefficient is a parametric procedure that puts into quantitative terms the association implied by a scatterplot of the two variables. For nonparametric data, use the Spearman's rank correlation.

89. Simple linear regression is a modeling method for determining the "best fit" linear equation formed between two sets of paired continuous data. The independent variable x and the dependent variable y form a line with slope m and y-intercept b:

$$y = mx + b$$

   A value of y can be predicted for a given value of x with variable accuracy, depending on the goodness of fit of the model.

90. The chi-square statistic is a nonparametric test of bivariate count or frequency data; it examines the disparity between the actual count frequencies and the expected count frequencies when a null hypothesis is true. For the determined degrees of freedom, a *p*-value is calculated, which indicates the probability of obtaining the observed chi-square value by chance alone. The higher the chi-square value, the less likely it is that chance is the cause of the distribution.

91. For typical regression analysis, the dependent variable must be continuous. Unless special techniques are used, the dependent variable must also be normally distributed and have variability that stays the same for all values of the independent variable.

92. The coefficient of determination (R^2) describes a regression model's goodness of fit as the proportion of the variation in the dependent variable (i.e., explained variation / total variation, ranging from 0 to 1) that the model explains. The closer R^2 is to1, the better the model explains the variation.

93. A logit coefficient (e.g., *expb*) can be interpreted as an odds ratio that tells the relative amount by which the overall odds ratio changes when the value of the independent variable x is increased by 1 unit.

94. The F statistic is used in analysis of variation between groups (ANOVA) and has two degrees of freedom: one for between-group variance and one for within-group variance. Reject the null hypothesis, if the F-ratio is much greater than 1.

95. The Cox proportional hazards model is a form of multivariable regression model used to analyze survival curves (e.g., Kaplan-Meier) and also clinical trials with a dichotomous outcome over time (e.g., dead vs. alive; diseased vs. disease-free).

96. Survival analysis is a statistical method for studying the time between an entry into a study and a subsequent event. Unequal observation time through censoring of the subjects under study makes survival analysis unique. Survival analysis is useful in making predictions about a population, comparing the effect of treatment between two groups, and investigating the importance of specific characteristics on survival.

97. A survival function, mathematically defined as $S(t) = P(T > t)$, describes the proportion of subjects surviving until or beyond a given time *t*.

98. The conditional failure rate, or hazard function, gives the instantaneous potential for failing at time *t* per unit of time, given survival up to time *t*.

99. The life table analysis divides the total period over which a group is observed into fixed intervals, giving an indication of the distribution of failures over time.

100. The Kaplan-Meier method allows the estimation of the survival function directly from the continuous survival or failure times. It provides for calculating the proportion surviving to each point in time that a failure or event occurs, rather than at fixed intervals, and generates a characteristic "stair step" survival curve.

CHAPTER 1

EPIDEMIOLOGY: AN HISTORICAL PERSPECTIVE

John L. Kane, MD

1. **Where can one find the earliest reference to epidemiologic thinking?**
   Hippocrates penned a tract called *On Airs, Waters, and Places* around 400 BC. He emphasized familiarity not only with the patients' symptoms, but also with the season of the year and the patients' living conditions, diet, fluid intake, and exercise habits:

   > For if one knows all these things well, or at least the greater part of them, he cannot miss knowing, when he comes into a strange city, either the diseases peculiar to the place, or the particular nature of common diseases, so that he will not be in doubt as to the treatment of the diseases, or commit mistakes, as is likely to be the case provided one had not previously considered these matters. And in particular, as the season and the year advances, he can tell what epidemic diseases will attack the city, either in summer or in winter, and what each individual will be in danger of experiencing from the change of regimen.

   Hippocrates: On Airs, Waters, and Places, Parts 1 and 2. Adams F (trans). 400 BC, Available at www.classics.mit.edu/Hippocrates/airwatpl.html.

2. **Who described wounds as "windows to the body"?**
   Galen, the great second century physician and anatomist, spent his early medical years as the surgeon to the gladiators in Pergamon. He employed as many as 20 scribes to write down all that he said in his work. Galen dissected countless animals in his prolific medical research. He also studied philosophy and wrote that a motive of profit was incompatible with a serious devotion to medicine, stating that doctors must learn to despise money. He was a proponent of the miasma theory of infection, which essentially blamed infection on clouds of poisonous gases.

   Galen. Available at http://www.med.virginia.edu/hs-library/historical/antiqua/galen.htm.

3. **What are the types of plague?**
   - Pulmonic: manifested by respiratory distress, pulmonary hemorrhage, and 100% mortality rate, it spreads easily through the air via respiratory secretions
   - Septicemic: often manifested by sudden death, without prior warning, after preferentially invading the bloodstream
   - Bubonic: manifested by the lymph node swelling on a large scale with cutaneous hemorrhage; approximately 60% of its victims died

4. **How many pandemics of plague have there been?**
   There have been three:
   - The first pandemic lasted from 541 to 544 AD and started in Pelusium, Egypt, before spreading throughout the Middle East and the Mediterranean basin. Accurate death statistics from this pandemic are not available. It is called the Justinian Plague because the Emperor Justinian succumbed to the disease.
   - The second pandemic, which decimated Europe and was called the Black Death, probably started in Sicily in 1347 and lasted until 1351. This plague likely came to Sicily from the Orient, spreading via shipping routes.

■ The third pandemic started in 1855 in the Chinese province of Yunnan and spread to the rest of the world, but especially devastated India and China. In India alone a total of 12.5 million people died.

Perry RD, Fetherston JD: *Yersinia pestis*—Etiologic agent of plague. Clin Microbiol Rev 10(1):35–66, 1997.

5. **How many people died from the Black Death?**
Exact numbers are not available, but estimates range from 17 to 28 million deaths, or about one-third of the European population, from 1330 to 1351.

6. **Are there any good literary descriptions of the bubonic plague?**
There are many. Two of particular note are *The Decameron* by Boccacio and *A Journal of the Plague Year* by Daniel Defoe (famous for *Moll Flanders* and *Robinson Crusoe*). *The Decameron* was written circa 1348 and describes the escape of seven men and three women from the ravages of the disease. Its author lived through the 1347 plague in Florence.

Defoe's book describes the plague in London in the year 1665, just before London's great fire. Defoe described the disease as follows:

> The Pain of the Swelling was in particular very violent, and to some intolerable; the Physicians and Surgeons may be said to have tortured many poor Creatures, even to Death. The Swellings in some grew hard, and they apply'd violent drawing Plasters, or Pultices, to break them; and if these did not do, they cut and scarified them in a terrible Manner: In some, those Swellings were made hard, partly by the Force of the Distemper, and partly by their being too violently drawn, and were so hard, that no Instrument could cut them and then they burnt them with Causticks, so that many died raving mad with the Torment; and some in the very Operation. . . . if these Swellings could be brought to a Head, and to break and run, or as the Surgeons call it, to digest, the Patient generally recover'd.

Defoe D: A Journal of the Plague Year. 1722. Oxford, Oxford University Press, 1990, pp 81–82.
Boccacio G: The Decameron of Giovanni Boccacio. Rigg JM (trans), c 1350. Available at http://www.brown.edu/Departments/Italian_Studies/dweb/dweb.shtml.

7. **What were the prevailing assumptions about the cause of the plague?**
The Paris Faculty of Medicine blamed the alignment of Saturn, Jupiter, and Mars that had occurred during March 1345. Others blamed comets and other stars. Some blamed the earthquake of 1348, saying it had released corrupting gases from below. Some blamed miasmas. And some noted that cities were hardest hit and postulated about various possibilities of contagions. Dr. Joseph Browne stated in his *Treatise on the Plague* that contagion is spread by "Air, diseased Persons, Goods transported from infected Places . . . Diet and Diseases that are the Causes of other Diseases."

Primarily, however, the plague was viewed as a curse from God, and many tried to identify the collective sin for which they were being punished. Unfortunately, much of the population blamed Jews, thinking that they were either actively poisoning the ground or water, or perhaps were bringing God's punishment simply by existing. In 1349 in Strasbourg, France, 2000 Jews were burned to death, and in Mainz, Germany, 6000 were incinerated. There are over 350 recorded massacres of the Jews during these years.

Browne J: A Practical Treatise of the Plague. 1720. Available at http://whqlibdoc.who.int/rare-books/a56989.pdf.

8. **What is the actual cause of plague?**
Infection with *Yersinia pestis*. The bacillus infects rats, causing their deaths. Fleas feeding on the rats' blood ingest the bacteria. When a host dies, the fleas jump to and infect the nearest available host, often human. Conditions in the Middle Ages, such as a large population of rats, wooden and thatched housing which allowed rats a ready entrance, and general overcrowding,

led to an easy spread of the disease. In 1894, during the third pandemic, the bacterium was discovered independently by two researchers, Shibasaburo Kitasato and Alexander Yersin, who called it *Pasteurella pestis* and linked it with the black rat. In 1897, Paul Louis Simond and Masanoro Gata (again independently) discovered the role of the flea in transmission.

Perry RD, Fetherston JD: *Yersinia pestis*—Etiologic Agent of Plague. Clin Microbiol Rev, 10(1):35–66, 1997.

9. **What measures were instituted to halt the spread of plague?**
The primary measure was isolation. As soon as plague was discovered in a house, the house was sealed and no one was allowed to enter or leave. Watchmen were posted to prevent occupants from venturing outside, often resulting in the deaths of entire households. Other measures included burning incense, ringing church bells or firing cannons, bathing in human urine, placing "stinks" (dead animals) in the home, employing leeches and other bloodletting, drinking the discharge from a bubo, drinking liquid gold, and the flagellant movement.

10. **Who were the flagellants?**
A group of dedicated religious men who walked from town to town in Europe in solitary processions lasting 33⅓ days. During their processions, they would gather in town squares and would beat themselves and others in their group with leather thongs tipped with metal pieces in the hope of purging themselves and the townspeople of their collective sin and guilt, thus turning aside God's wrath, which had descended in the form of the plague. The gatherings were attended by much emotion and often led to persecution of local Jews. The pope initially approved of the movement, but it fell rather quickly into papal disfavor; the movement vanished in 1350.

KEY POINTS: IMPORTANT DATES

1. 400 BC: Hippocrates published "On Airs, Waters, and Places," which presented the epidemiologic principles of the observation and recording of patients' habits, diets, and environments in the prediction of disease patterns.

2. 1747: James Lind did a randomized, controlled trial to establish the cause of scurvy.

3. 1946: CDC established from the Office of Malaria Control in War Areas.

4. 1977: The last naturally occurring case of smallpox was diagnosed in a Somali man.

11. **Who is John Graunt?**
A self-educated London businessman who, around 1620, noted the wealth of potentially important information available in London's *Weekly Bills of Mortality*. Graunt began collecting and tabulating the data. In 1662, he published *Natural and Political Observations,* based on his examination of the *Bills of Mortality*. This was the first use and publication of a record of vital statistics.

12. **What were some of Graunt's findings?**
Graunt noted that a true count of plague deaths could not be kept without a meticulous reckoning of deaths from the numerous other diseases of the day. He observed that one third of liveborn infants died before age 5, 2 people of every 9 died of acute disease, and 70 out of 229 died of chronic disease. He also noted that 7% of the population died of age and that only 1 in 4000 died of starvation in London.

In addition, Graunt made observations and suggestions about the employment of beggars, the morality of suicide, and whether making gold would benefit the population.

Graunt J: Natural and Political Observations Mentioned in a following Index, and made upon the Bills of Mortality. 1622. Available at http://www.ac.wwu.edu/~stephan/Graunt/bills.html.

13. **Who was called the English Hippocrates?**

Thomas Sydenham (1624–1689) bears this epithet. He was an English physician who revived the practice of Hippocrates by reemphasizing detailed clinical observation. Sydenham believed that the study of medicine was at the patients' bedsides. He is considered a father of epidemiology and contributed treatises on gout, malaria, scarlatina, measles, hysteria, and the post-streptococcal nervous disorder that bears his name, Sydenham's chorea. He was quoted as saying, "The arrival of a good clown exercises a more beneficial influence upon the health of a town than of twenty asses laden with drugs."

Thomas Sydenham. Available at http://www.whonamedit.com.

14. **What does De Morbis Artificum Diatriba describe?**

Written by Ramazzini and published in 1700, it is the first comprehensive work about occupational diseases. It describes the health hazards encountered by workers in 52 occupations, including masons, farmers, nurses, and soldiers. Ramazzini discussed the difficulties faced by "learned men" from overtaxed minds, as well as the need for cleanliness among midwives and the dangers of contracting syphilitic infection.

Bernardino Ramazzini. Available at http://www.whonamedit.com.

15. **What is scurvy?**

Scurvy is a vitamin C deficiency that results in the breakdown of collagen and leads, among other manifestations, to a lack of collagen in the walls of capillaries, causing hemorrhaging in cells throughout the body. The patient becomes weak and has joint pain secondary to periosteal bleeding. Raised red spots appear on the skin around the hair follicles of the legs, buttocks, arms, and back. Gums hemorrhage, and their tissue becomes weak and spongy. Dentin, which lies below the enamel and is part of the root of teeth, breaks down. Teeth loosen, and eating becomes difficult and painful.

16. **How was scurvy described by a nonmedical observer?**

Richard Walter, a chaplain in the Royal Navy during a 1740 voyage, described the symptoms including skin black as ink, ulcers, difficult respiration, rictus of the limbs, teeth falling out, and, perhaps most revolting of all, a strange plethora of gum tissue sprouting out of the mouth, which immediately rotted and lent the victim's breath an abominable odor.

Lamb J: Captain Cook and the Scourge of Scurvy. 2002. Available at http://www.bbc.co.uk/history/discovery/exploration/captaincook_scurvy_01.shtml.

17. **Why did scurvy become a problem only with long voyages?**

The deficiency takes 2–6 months to manifest symptoms and the symptoms can be improved with the consumption of vitamin C, which the sailors ate voraciously when in port. Vasco da Gama lost two-thirds of his crew to the disease while making his way to India in 1499, and Magellan lost more than 80% while crossing the Pacific Ocean.

18. **Why did the Vikings not get scurvy on their long voyages?**

The Vikings ate cloudberry and a plant called *Skjørbuksurt* (i.e., scurvygrass or *Cochleria officinalis*), both rich sources of vitamin C.

19. **What is one of the first recorded randomized clinical trials?**

In 1747, James Lind, a Scottish physician in the Royal Navy, selected 12 patients with scurvy and fed them a variety of diets. Two received cider, two received elixir of vitriol, two received vinegar, two received seawater, two received lemons and oranges, and two received purgatives. One of the patients receiving the citrus fruit was fit for duty within 6 days, and the other was well enough to nurse the remainder of the patients. The only other patients who showed any improvement were those who drank the cider, but improvement was only slight. Despite this success, the British Admiralty took 50 years before it required citrus to be available on all of its ships.

Lind J: A Treatise of the Scurvy in Three Parts. Containing an inquiry into the Nature, Causes and Cure of that Disease, together with a Critical and Chronological View of what has been published on the subject. London, A. Millar, 1753. Available at http://www.people.virginia.edu/~rjh9u/scurvy.html.

20. **What is Devonshire colic?**
Lead poisoning. From 1762–1767, almost 300 cases of the disease were taken to Exeter hospitals. George Baker, an English physician, noted that the symptoms were similar to those found in painters with lead poisoning. He discovered that Devonshire cider contained lead and that cider presses there, unlike presses in the rest of the country, were lined with sheets of lead.

KEY POINTS: IMPORTANT PEOPLE

1. John Graunt: began the collection and analysis of the *Weekly Bills of Mortality* in London in the 1600s, showing the value of a system of disease surveillance

2. Edward Jenner: developed and tested an immunization for smallpox

3. P. C. A. Louis: called "the father of modern clinical epidemiology," he was responsible for the landmark study of the noneffectiveness of bloodletting

4. Ignac Semmelweis: dramatically reduced the rate of childbed fever by the institution of handwashing

21. **What was the medical burden of smallpox in the 18th century?**
An estimated 400,000 deaths resulted from infection with smallpox worldwide, and of those who survived, one third were blinded by corneal infection. In addition, survivors were deeply scarred with pockmarks. Patients were known to be immune once they had contracted and survived smallpox.

22. **How was the knowledge of lifelong immunity to smallpox after infection used in an effort to prevent disease?**
A process called *variolation* was used. Healthy people were given material from the lesions of patients with smallpox. Unfortunately, this method resulted in deaths from smallpox and infected other patients.

23. **What did dairy maids have to do with developing a vaccine to smallpox?**
In 1768, Edward Jenner overheard a dairymaid who claimed, "I can't take the smallpox, for I have already had the cowpox." He observed that dairymaids who had suffered the milder cowpox infection were indeed immune to smallpox outbreaks.

24. **What did Jenner do with this knowledge?**
To test the hypothesis, Jenner took the exudate from a cowpox pustule on the hand of dairymaid Sarah Nelmes and injected it into the skin of 8-year-old James Phipps (Fig. 1-1). Six weeks later, Jenner administered material from a fresh smallpox pustule into young James and the boy did not contract the disease.

25. **In relation to smallpox, who could be described as the unluckiest person on the planet?**
The last naturally occurring case of smallpox occurred in a Somali man in 1977. The World Health Organization declared smallpox eradicated in 1980. Interestingly, Jenner's experiments were guided entirely by observation. The prevailing theory of disease was still the miasmatic

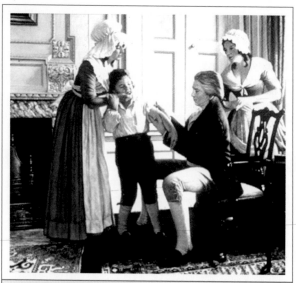

Figure 1-1. Painting by Robert A. Thom of the first vaccination, performed by Edward Jenner on May 14, 1796, in his apartment in the Chantry House, Berkeley, Gloucestershire (From Great Moments in Medicine. Parke-Davis & Company, 1966. Courtesy of Parke-Davis & Company.)

concept, which held that disease was transmitted by a miasma, or cloud, which clung low on the surface of the earth. Jenner had no knowledge of viruses or bacteria.

Gordis L: Epidemiology, 2nd ed. Philadelphia, W.B. Saunders, 2000, pp 9–11.

26. **What peculiar type of cancer did Sir Percival Potts link to the occupation of chimney sweep circa 1775?**
    Sir Percival Potts was an English surgeon who identified a high rate of scrotal cancer in chimney sweeps. Potts described the cancer as follows:

    > It is a disease which always makes its first attack on, and its first appearance in, the inferior part of the scrotum; where it produces a superficial, painful, ragged, ill-looking sore, with hard and rising edges: the trade call it the soot-wart. I never saw it under the age of puberty, which is, I suppose, one reason why it is generally taken, both by patient and surgeon, for venereal; and being treated with mercurials, is thereby soon and much exasperated.

    Potts surmised that the soot collecting in the folds of the scrotum was the causative agent and thus become an early identifier of occupational cancer risk.

    Percival PS: Chirurgical Observations Relative to the Polypus of the Nose, the Cancer of the Scrotum, the Different Kinds of Ruptures, and the Mortification of the Toes and Feet. London, Hawes, Clarke, & Collins, 1775.

27. **Why did scrotal cancer rates decrease significantly in Danish chimney workers after this finding, while the English rates stayed the same?**
    The Danish government began requiring its workers to wear protective clothing and to bathe regularly. The British continued to bathe only once each week for many years after Potts's report.

28. **What does wine-making have to do with the germ theory?**
    During his study of the fermentation of wine, Louis Pasteur, a French chemist, proved the process was caused by microorganisms from the environment, which were transmitted to the

liquid via dust particles and not by spontaneous generation within the wine itself. Pasteur's experiments finally disproved conclusively the theory that life could arise spontaneously in organic materials, a theory that had been scientific dogma for over 200 years.

Louis Pasteur, Embassy of France in Canada. Available at http://www.ambafrance-ca.org.

29. **How did Robert Koch advance the germ theory?**
He established Koch's postulates, as follows:
- The causative agent must be present in every case of the disease and must not be present in healthy animals.
- The pathogen must be isolated from the diseased host animal and must be grown in pure culture.
- The same disease must be produced when microbes from the pure culture are inoculated into healthy, susceptible animals.
- The same pathogen must be recoverable once again from this artificially infected animal and must be able to be grown in pure culture.

Wubah DA: The Germ Theory of Disease. Available at http://www.towson.edu/~wubah/medmicro/ Germ_theory.htm.

30. **Who is often called "the father of modern clinical epidemiology"? Why?**
P. C. A. Louis (1787–1872), who designed and performed an experiment to assess whether bloodletting for inflammatory conditions conferred any medical benefit. Louis lived during a time when leading medical authorities, such as Francois Joseph Broussais in Paris, considered inflammation to be the cause of all diseases. J. J. Jackson, another prominent physician, wrote in 1836 that "if anything may be regarded as settled in the treatment of diseases, it is that bloodletting is useful in the class of diseases called inflammatory; and especially in inflammations of the thoracic viscera." France imported 42 million leeches in 1833.

Morabia A: P. C. A. Louis and the birth of clinical epidemiology. J Clin Epidemiol 49 (12):1327–1333, 1996.

KEY POINTS: IMPORTANT PLACES

1. Broad Street, London: site of John Snow's important research on cholera.
2. Cuba (1898): Walter Reed conducted important research on yellow fever.
3. Tuskegee, Alabama: site of the infamous "Tuskegee Study of Untreated Syphilis in the Negro Male."
4. Framingham, Massachusetts: site of the Framingham Heart Study.

31. **How did Louis conduct the study?**
He performed a case-controlled study. He selected 77 patients who had been admitted to the hospital with pneumonia and did a chart review. After controlling for other confounding factors such as age, gender, and severity of illness, he compared the effect of early (days 1-4) versus late bloodletting (days 5 to recovery or death) on the duration and outcome of the pneumonia. All of the patients were in perfect health at the onset of the disease.

32. **What were the results?**
The disease lasted 17.7 days in the early bleeding group and 20.3 days in the late bleeding group. Risk of death was 44% in the early group versus 25% in the late group. Louis described this as "a startling and apparently absurd result." Overall, he concluded that the effect of bloodletting was "much less than has been commonly believed." Over the next 15 years, leech imports fell to a few thousand per year.

Hadjiliadis D: Early clinical statistics. Available at http://www.med.unc.edu/wrkunits/syllabus/yr4/gen/medhist/publish/earlyclinstats.ppt.

Morabia A: P. C. A. Louis and the birth of clinical epidemiology. J Clin Epidemiol 49 (12):1327–1333, 1996.

33. **What society was formed with the mission to "collect, preserve, and diffuse statistical information in the different departments of human knowledge?"**
The American Statistical Society, which was formed in Boston in 1839 by William Cogswell, Richard Fletcher, John Dix Fisher, Oliver Peabody, and Lemuel Shattuck. In 1840, the name was changed to the American Statistical Association. One of its early members was Florence Nightingale.

The American Statistical Association at http://www.amstat.org/about/index.cfm?fuseaction=history

34. **What was the origin of the National Institutes of Health?**
A one-room facility within the Marine Hospital on Staten Island, New York, called the Laboratory of Hygiene, was established in 1887. Dr. Joseph Kinyoun was the director and sole employee of this, the government's first research facility. It was later renamed the Hygienic Laboratory and relocated to Washington DC. In 1930, with the passing of the Ransdell Act, the title of National Institutes of Health (NIH) was adopted. The NIH grew in scope and size and was moved to Bethesda, Maryland, in 1938.

35. **Where is Broad Street?**
Located in London, Broad Street was made infamous in 1855 by its cholera-tainted water pump.

36. **Who was the anesthesiologist who administered chloroform to Queen Victoria during the birth of her children? What does this have to do with Broad Street?**
John Snow was highly interested in the epidemiology of cholera. Deaths from cholera in London in the 1800s were high, and Snow believed that the cause of cholera was a sort of poison that the infected person excreted in his feces and vomitus, and that healthy patients contracted the disease by ingesting water that had been contaminated with the vomit or feces of cholera patients.

The Registrar General, William Farr, disagreed with Snow's theory. Farr subscribed to the miasmatic theory of disease, which held that a cloud of infection clinging close to the ground spread disease. One could theoretically escape infection by going to higher altitudes. Farr tabulated statistics showing that patients living at higher altitudes had less risk of contracting cholera.

Snow observed the cluster of cholera deaths in the geographic area supplied by the Broad Street pump, which was supplied by the Southwark and Vauxhaul Company, whereas the Lambeth Company supplied water to other city locations. Both companies extracted their water supplies from the Thames River, but the intake for the Southwark Company was in a highly polluted part of the river, while the Lambeth Company had recently shifted its intake upstream to a less polluted part of the river. Snow traced the water supply for the cholera victims and was able to show that the death rate from cholera was almost 10 times higher in houses that received water from the Southwark Company (Fig. 1-2).

Gordis L: Epidemiology, 2nd ed. Philadelphia, W. B. Saunders, 2000, pp 10–11.

37. **What is childbed fever?**
Also known as puerperal sepsis, it is an aggressive infection occurring after delivery of a child. It claimed the life of Jane Seymour, third wife of Henry VIII, as well as Mary Wollstonecraft, the mother of Mary Shelley. In the 1700s it claimed the lives of as many as 20% of new mothers.

38. **How does hand-washing relate to childbed fever?**
Ignac Semmelweis (1813–1865) found that simply washing hands before examining mothers-to-be could virtually eliminate this illness. He worked at a maternity hospital and noticed that the

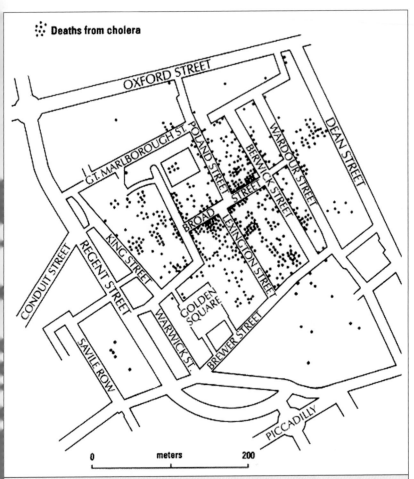

Deaths from cholera

Figure 1-2. Map of cholera deaths in London. (From http://www.nationalgeographic.com/resources/ngo/education/ideas912/912choleraho1.html, with permission.)

rate of death was higher among women who delivered in the hospital than among those who had given birth at home en route to the hospital. He also noted that women who delivered prematurely became ill less frequently. He noted that at times a whole row of beds would die of childbed fever.

Mothers-to-be would beg not to be admitted to the first division, where students and doctors practiced. Patients desired admission to the second division where midwives performed the deliveries. Semmelweis studied the meticulous record-keeping and confirmed that death rates in the first division were often 12 times those of the second division. He ensured that all deliveries in the first and second division were done from the lateral position in order to standardize his environment. This strategy did not affect the death rate.

39. **How did Semmelweis unravel the childbed fever conundrum?**
A professor was pricked with a knife used at autopsy and developed an ascending infection that subsequently took his life. Semmelweis noted that the disease seemed identical to the disease

that had afflicted so many maternity patients. Autopsies of the women and their newborns confirmed that the disease was indeed the same that had affected the professor.

The medical students at this school were highly encouraged to do anatomic studies with the cadavers, and hand-washing was not performed between dissections and the examination and delivery of maternity patients. In May 1847, chlorine washings were introduced, reducing the number of maternal deaths to a level below that of the second division.

Caplan, CE: The Childbed Fever Mystery and the Meaning of Medical Journalism. Available at http://www.med.mcgill.ca/mjm/issues/v01n01/fever.html.

40. **What is yellow fever?**
A viral hemorrhagic fever caused by the yellow fever virus, which is transmitted to humans from the bite of an infected *Aedes aegypti* mosquito. The liver, heart, kidneys, and lymphoid tissue are attacked, and the skin becomes icteric—hence, the "yellow."

KEY POINTS: IMPORTANT DISEASES

1. Plague: killed one third of Europe's population in the Middle Ages

2. Scurvy: the scourge of sailors, it limited the distance that ships could travel

3. Smallpox: caused approximately 400,000 deaths in the 18th century and blinded 33% of survivors

4. AIDS: the modern plague, AIDS ended the sexual revolution

41. **Which war acted as a stimulant to solving the riddle of yellow fever?**
The Spanish-American War of 1898 featured a yellow fever epidemic in Cuba early in the war. The U.S. Surgeon General sent a team of researchers led by army medical scientist Walter Reed. Many ideas were tested in the field, including a 50-year-old theory proposed by Dr. Carlos Finlay that yellow fever might be spread by insects. Reed divided a group of volunteers into two groups. The first slept on the contaminated clothes and bed linens of yellow fever patients but were protected by mosquito netting; the second slept on clean linens but were without netting. The patients who were protected by the netting did not contract yellow fever, but the others did. This discovery led to the widespread use of protective mosquito netting and, consequently, to a monumental reduction in the occurrence of yellow fever.

Marton, T: Yellow Fever and Dr. Walter Reed, 1999. Available at http://www.mcatmaster.com/medicine&war/yellowfever.htm.

42. **What is another name for enteric fever?**
Typhoid fever, which is unique to humans, causing fevers as high as 104°F malaise, abdominal discomfort, rose spot rash, splenomegaly, and leukopenia. The gravest complications are intestinal hemorrhage and perforation. It is caused by the bacteria *Salmonella typhi* and is transmitted to others through the fecal-oral route.

43. **What does the Clergy Orphans' School in St. John's Wood have to do with typhoid fever?**
An outbreak of typhoid fever occurred there in 1856, affecting many of the young students. A letter to the *Lancet* described the outbreak. The first pupil took ill on September 14; that pupil was followed by four other cases over the ensuing 3 weeks, and then 19 cases within a 36-hour period. The patients suffered fever, lassitude, diarrhea, and a papular rash. Because of the

simultaneous onset in this group, the author believed that the outbreak could not be attributed to a contagion: "The simultaneous seizure of the patients is sufficient to set aside the idea of contagion. Some local cause was, obviously, at work."

44. What response was generated by this letter?
William Budd responded with a well-reasoned letter, clearly showing that the symptoms described were very consistent with typhoid. Budd theorized that the diarrhea from the infected patients contained a concentrated poison which, when ingested by a healthy person, would make him ill. He postulated that the diarrhea had percolated through the earth to the nearby well, which thereby acted as the source of the larger outbreak. Budd continued to write about typhoid, eventually publishing *Typhoid Fever, Its Nature, Mode of Spreading and Prevention* in March of 1873.

Budd W: Typhoid Fever, its Nature, Mode of Spreading and Prevention. 1873, Appendix. Available at http://www.deltaomega.org/typhoid.pdf.

45. Who is Mary Mallon?
Mary Mallon was born in Ireland in 1869 and immigrated to America in 1884 at age 15. She found work as a cook in New York City. In that capacity she infected 47 people with typhoid fever, 3 of whom died. She became well-known as Typhoid Mary. In the summer of 1906, banker Charles Henry Warren took his family on vacation to Long Island, bringing Mary as his cook. Of the 11 residents at the house, 6 became ill with typhoid. The owner of the house hired civil engineer George Soper to trace the source of typhoid, fearing that it might be from his home. Soper traced it to Mallon and also found that, in the seven jobs she had held since 1900, there had been 22 cases of typhoid and 1 death. Mallon was the first patient to be found carrying typhoid without suffering from the disease.

46. How did Mary Mallon respond to the news of her carrier status?
When Soper approached her to request blood, urine, and fecal samples, she seized a kitchen knife and chased him from her house. He returned later with reinforcements, including the police. Mallon met them at the door with a long fork, lunged at them, and, in the confusion, ran into the interior of the house. After a 5-hour search, they finally found her hidden in a closet.

47. What did the health department do with Mary?
After she was confirmed to be a carrier, she was taken to an isolated cottage on North Brother Island near the Bronx.

48. When was she allowed to return to New York City?
In 1910, when a new public health commissioner took over, Mary was released on the condition that she promised not to take any employment that required cooking. She also had to come to the health department on a regular basis for retesting.

49. Who was Mary Brown?
She was a cook employed at the Sloane Maternity Hospital in Manhattan, where in January of 1915 an outbreak of typhoid fever affected 25 people, 2 of whom died. Her real name was Mary Mallon. She lived the rest of her live on North Brother Island in the isolated cottage, suffering a stroke in 1932 and dying in 1938.

Rosenberg J: Typhoid Mary. Available at http://history1900s.about.com/library/weekly/aa062900a.htm.

50. What causes pellagra?
A deficiency of niacin. Pellagra is a disease with prominent skin symptoms that can be mistaken for leprosy. Other symptoms include dementia and diarrhea. Prevailing thought early in the 20th century was that pellagra was transmitted by bacteria.

KEY POINTS: HOW TO WIN A BET IN A BAR FREQUENTED BY EPIDEMIOLOGISTS

1. Typhoid Mary's name: Mary Mallon.

2. Devonshire colic: lead poisoning contracted from drinking cider made in Devonshire, where the presses were lined with sheets of lead.

3. Soot-wart: the name for scrotal cancer common in chimney sweeps in London in the 1700s.

4. Gaetan Dugas: A Canadian airline steward falsely thought to be the initial case of AIDS in the United States.

---

51. Why did Joseph Goldberger disagree with the germ theory of pellagra?

He noted that only inmates contracted the disease in the Southern asylums and orphanages. An infectious source would affect the staff as well, and this pattern never occurred. He theorized and ultimately proved that dietary deficiencies were the cause.

Dr. Joseph Goldberg and the War on Pellagra. Available at http://history.nih.gov/exhibits/goldberger/docs/pellegra_5.htm.

52. What is the Tuskegee study?

The Public Health Service, in conjunction with the Tuskegee Institute, began a study in 1932 in Macon County, Alabama, called "The Tuskegee Study of Untreated Syphilis in the Negro Male." The men were informed that they were being treated for "bad blood." There were 600 patients, 399 with syphilis and 201 without the disease. The study lasted 40 years, despite having been originally designed to last 6 months. Penicillin was known to cure syphilis by 1947, but the men in the study were not offered the treatment, and there was no evidence that they were informed that they could quit the study if they desired. The *New York Times* broke the story in 1972.

The Tuskegee Syphilis Study: A Hard Lesson Learned. Available at http://www.cdc.gov/nchstp/od/tuskegee/time.htm.

53. When was the Centers for Disease Control and Prevention (CDC) established?

The Office of Malaria Control in War Areas was in place during World War II and given the task of malaria control in the southeastern United States. The Center for Communicable Diseases was established in 1946 as a successor to this office. After malaria was eliminated in the United States, the CDC greatly expanded its public health role, changing its name to Centers for Disease Control in 1970, with the phrase "and Prevention" added in 1992.

Malaria, CDC Origins. Available at http://www.cdc.gov.

54. Why is Natick, Massachusetts, almost famous in the history of epidemiology?

It is the town closest to Framingham, where the Framingham study was begun in 1948 to study the risk factors for heart disease. This study was a long-term observational study that initially involved 5127 people, aged 30–62 years, who showed no signs of heart disease. The participants were evaluated with questionnaires and a physical exam every other year for 30 years. Many of the basics of our understanding of coronary artery disease came from this study.

Framingham Heart Study. Available at http://www.clinicaltrials.gov/show/NCT00005121.

55. When was the link between cigarette smoking and lung cancer first noticed?

In 1950, two researchers presented data that showed a link between cigarette smoking and lung cancer. The first was named Ernst Wynder, who became interested in the link after witnessing an autopsy of a smoker and noting the blackness of the lungs. He interviewed patients with lung cancer and patients with other cancers and found a much higher incidence of lung cancer in the smokers. The other researcher was a British scientist who interviewed numerous physicians about their smoking habits and then watched to see who developed lung cancer. He again demonstrated a link.

Does smoking really cause lung cancer? Dr. George Johnson, On Science. Available at http://www.txtwriter.com/Onscience/Articles/smokingcancer.html.

56. What was the Lalonde Report?

It was a 1974 report entitled *A New Perspective on the Health of Canadians*. The report was groundbreaking because it de-emphasized the importance of biomedical interventions in the individual well-being of people and instead identified four areas that were primarily responsible for patient health: environment, human biology, lifestyle, and health care organization.

Lalonde M: A New Perspective on the Health of Canadians, a working document. 1974. Available at http://www.hc-sc.gc.ca/hppb/phdd/pdf/perspective.pdf.

57. What product's motto was "It even absorbs the worry"?

Rely tampons. In 1980, 55 cases of a newly described disease called toxic shock syndrome were reported to the CDC. The symptoms consisted of high fever, sunburn-like rash, desquamation, hypotension, and multiorgan system damage. Women accounted for 52 of the 55 cases, and case-controlled studies indicated a high association with tampon use. Subsequent studies traced the highest risk to users of Rely tampons, which were a particularly high absorbency tampon.

Centers for Disease Control: Historical Perspectives Reduced Incidence of Menstrual Toxic-Shock Syndrome—United States 1980–1990. MMWR 39(25):421–423, 1990.

58. When did acquired immunodeficiency syndrome (AIDS) come to public attention?

The *Morbidity and Mortality Weekly Report* (MMWR) published an article called *Pneumocystis Pneumonia—Los Angeles* on June 5, 1981, describing five cases of pneumocystis pneumonia in active homosexuals. Two of the patients died and all five were infected with cytomegalovirus (CMV) and oral candidiasis. The concluding paragraph reads:

> All the above observations suggest the possibility of a cellular-immune dysfunction related to a common exposure that predisposes individuals to opportunistic infections such as pneumocystosis and candidiasis. Although the role of CMV infection in the pathogenesis of pneumocystosis remains unknown, the possibility of *P. carinii* infection must be carefully considered in a differential diagnosis for previously healthy homosexual males with dyspnea and pneumonia.

Centers for Disease Control: Pneumocystic pneumonia—Los Angeles. MMWR 37(12):81, 1981.

59. Who was the first patient to introduce AIDS to the United States?

This question does not have a known answer. Patient Zero, Gaetan Dugas, was mistakenly thought to be this index patient. He was identified by the CDC as Patient Zero in an early epidemiologic study, in which 40 of 228 patients diagnosed with AIDS by April 1992 had had sex with this Canadian airline steward. However, there had been numerous AIDS cases in the United States before Dugas.

Gaetan Dugas. The Free Dictionary. Available at www.encyclopedia.thefreedictionary.com.

60. What is the Muerto Canyon virus?

The virus is now better known as the *sin nombraue virus* and the etiologic agent in hantavirus pulmonary syndrome. The disease first came to light when a young, healthy Navajo man living in the southwestern United States became short of breath and rapidly died. His fiancée had died 2 days previously. Researchers documented numerous other cases, and the CDC's labs were able to pinpoint an unknown type of hantavirus.

Hantaviruses were known to be transported to humans from rodents, and testing revealed that the deer mouse was the main host. The spread was from aerosolized dried rodent feces inhaled by the human host. The reason for the outbreak in 1993 is thought to be a population explosion of the rodent population to 10 times their normal numbers. The area had been drought-stricken for many years, and then, in 1993, adequate rainfall revived plant life in the area and the mice had an abundant supply of food.

Tracking a Mystery Disease: The Detailed Story of Hantavirus Pulmonary Syndrome. Available at http://www.cdc.gov.

WEBSITES

1. http://www.classics.mit.edu/Hippocrates/airwatpl.html

2. http://www.med.virginia.edu/hs-library/historical/antiqua/galen.htm

3. http://www.brown.edu/Departments/Italian_Studies/dweb/dweb.shtml

4. http://www.whqlibdoc.who.int/rare-books/a56989.pdf

5. http://www.ac.wwu.edu/~stephan/Graunt/b.Us.html

6. http://www.whonamedit.com

7. http://www.bbc.co.uk/history/discovery/exploration/captaincook_scurvy_01.shtml

8. http://www.people.virginia.edu/~rjh9u/scurvy.html

9. http://www.ambafrance-ca.org

10. http://www.towson.edu/~wubah/medmicro/Germ_theory.htm

11. http://www.med.unc.edu/wrkunits/syllabus/yr4/gen/medhist/publish/earlyclinstats.ppt

12. http://www.med.mcgill.ca/mjm/issues/v01n01/fever.html

13. http://www.mcatmaster.com/medicine&war/yellowfever.htm

14. http://www.deltaomega.org/typhoid.pdf

15. http://www.history1900s.about.com/library/weekly/aa062900a.htm

16. http://www.history.nih.gov/exhibits/goldberger/docs/pellegra_5.htm

17. http://www.cdc.gov/nchstp/od/tuskegee/time.htm

18. http://www.cdc.gov

19. http://www.clinicaltrials.gov/show/NCT00005121

20. http://www.txtwriter.com/Onscience/Articles/smokingcancer.html

21. http://www.hc-sc.gc.ca/hppb/phdd/pdf/perspective.pdf

22. http://www.encyclopedia.thefreedictionary.com

23. http://www.amstat.org/about/index.cfm?fuseaction=history

BIBLIOGRAPHY

1. Centers for Disease Control: Historical perspectives reduced incidence of menstrual toxic-shock syndrome—United States 1980-1990. MMWR 39(25):421–433, 1990.

2. Centers for Disease Control: Pneumocystic pneumonia—Los Angeles. MMWR 37(12):81, 1981.

3. Defoe D: A Journal of the Plague Year [1722]. Oxford, Oxford University Press, 1990, pp 81–82.

4. Gordis L: Epidemiology, 2nd ed. Philadelphia, W.B. Saunders, 2000, pp 9-11.5. Morabia A: P. C. A. Louis and the birth of clinical epidemiology. J Clin Epidemiol 49(12):1327–1333, 1996.

5. Percival PS: Chirurgical Observations Relative to the Polypus of the Nose, the Cancer of the Scrotum, the Different Kinds of Ruptures, and the Mortification of the Toes and Feet. London, Hawes, Clarke, & Collins, 1775.

6. Perry RD, Fetherston JD: *Yersinia pestis*—Etiologic agent of plague. Clin Microbiol Rev 10(1):35–66, 1997.

CHAPTER 2

INTRODUCTION TO EPIDEMIOLOGIC PRINCIPLES

Patrick R. Laraby, MD, MBA, MPH

1. **What is epidemiology?**
   Epidemiology is the study of the distribution and determinates of disease in the human population. It is the basic science and fundamental practice of public health.

2. **Where does the word *epidemiology* come from?**
   The word *epidemiology* comes from *epidemic*, which, translated from Greek, means "upon the people."

3. **What do epidemiologists do?**
   Epidemiologists study disease frequencies in populations to identify risk factors for disease (and health) to ultimately improve the health of the population.

4. **What is health?**
   According to the World Health Association (WHO), health is a state of complete physical, mental, and social well-being, and not merely the absence of disease or infirmity.

5. **What is preventive medicine?**
   The application of preventive measures by clinical professionals to maintain health.

6. **What is public health?**
   The application of preventive medicine principles to a population.

7. **Describe the levels of prevention.**
   - Primary prevention: the prevention of disease or injury
   - Secondary prevention: the early detection and prompt treatment of disease
   - Tertiary prevention: the reduction of disability and the promotion of rehabilitation from disease

8. **What are Leavell's levels?**
   Hugh Leavell developed a user-friendly paradigm for preventive health that correlates stage of disease, level of prevention, and the appropriate response by health professionals. The levels are as follows:
   1. **Pre-disease**
      a. With no known risk factors: primary prevention should be health promotion (e.g., encouragement of healthy changes in lifestyle, nutrition, and environment).
      b. With disease susceptibility: primary prevention should include specific protection (e.g., recommendations for nutritional supplements, immunizations, and occupational and vehicle safety).
   2. **Latent disease:** secondary prevention should focus on screening for populations or case findings for the individual in medical care and, if disease is found, treatment.
   3. **Symptomatic disease**
      a. Initial care: tertiary prevention should focus on disability limitation (i.e., medical or surgical treatment to limit damage from the disease with primary prevention measures).

b. Subsequent care: tertiary prevention should focus on rehabilitation (i.e., teaching of methods to reduce social disability).

Leavell HR, Cark EG: Preventive Medicine for the Doctor in His Community, 3rd ed. New York, McGraw-Hill, 1965.

9. **Explain the goal of screening programs.**
Screening programs are a secondary prevention strategy used to identify diseases before they are symptomatic, as well as to institute a new treatment program to reduce morbidity and/or mortality.

10. **What are the two fundamental assumptions of epidemiology?**
   - Human disease does not occur at random.
   - Human disease has causal and preventive factors that can be identified through systematic investigation of different populations or population subgroups in varying places or times.

Hennekens CH: Epidemiology in Medicine. Boston, Little, Brown & Company, 1987.

11. **Who is John Snow?**
Modern epidemiologists view John Snow as arguably the greatest pioneer of their field. He detailed the facts about sources of drinking water that he related to mortality rates from cholera in London from 1853–1954. His work proved the classic demonstration of the mode of transmission of cholera long before *Vibrio* was identified.

12. **Explain the uses of epidemiology.**
The most important use of epidemiology is to improve our understanding of health and disease. Epidemiologist Jeremy Morris defined five uses of epidemiology:
   1. Historical study: determining whether community health is getting better or worse
   2. Community assessment: defining actual and potential health problems
   3. Working with health services: improving efficacy, effectiveness, and efficiency
   4. Individual risk and chances: determining actuary risk and health hazards appraisals for individuals and populations (e.g., What is the risk that an individual will die before his next birthday?)
   5. Completing the clinical picture: offering different presentations of a disease

Morris JN: Uses of Epidemiology, 3rd ed. Edinburgh, Churchill-Livingstone, 1975.

13. **Illustrate the epidemiologic sequence.**
An orderly sequence characterizes epidemiology and is best explained using an example, such as the association between lung cancer and cigarette smoking, as follows:
   1. **Observing:** scientific observation on smoking and cancer appeared in a few well-known publications in the 1920s.
   2. **Counting cases or events:** vital statistics trends showed an increase in deaths caused by lung cancer in the United States.
   3. **Relating cases or events to population at risk:** increased death rates from lung cancer were reported in national vital statistics in countries where smoking was an established lifestyle characteristic.
   4. **Making comparisons:** studies of British physicians in the 1950s provided definitive comparisons between smoking and lung cancer.
   5. **Developing a hypothesis:** because cigarette smoke contains more than 2500 chemical components, some of which are carcinogenic in animals, only a small logical step was required to go from inference to hypothesis.
   6. **Testing the hypothesis:** epidemiologic studies showed a consistent relationship between the present occurrence of lung cancer and a history of cigarette smoking with a dose-response relationship.

7. **Making scientific inferences:** observations led to valid scientific inferences about the association of tobacco smoking and lung cancer. These include (1) clinical observations, (2) national trends in mortality in countries with high cigarette smoking prevalence, (3) epidemiologic comparisons in large groups representing different segments of the national population in more than one country, and (4) the biologic effects of tobacco smoke. All of these observations led to the inference that smoking increased the risk of dying from lung cancer.

8. **Conducting experimental studies:** laboratory animal studies showed that exposure to tobacco smoke produces precancerous lesions followed by squamous cell carcinoma in both animals and humans.

9. **Intervening and evaluating:** action by public health agencies reduced the cigarette smoking rates. A decline in mortality trends in smoking-related causes follows this reduction.

Doll R, Hill AB: The mortality of doctors in relation to their smoking habits: A preliminary report. Br Med J 1:1451-1455, 1954.

14. **What does the term *descriptive epidemiology* mean?**
Descriptive epidemiology is concerned with describing the general characteristics of the distribution of disease, particularly in relation to person, place, and time. Descriptive data provide valuable information, enabling health care providers and administrators to allocate resources efficiently and to plan effective prevention and education programs.

15. **List the types of descriptive epidemiologic studies.**
- **Ecologic studies (i.e., correlation studies):** use data from entire populations to compare disease frequencies between different groups during the same period of time or in the same population at different points in time. These studies are useful for the formulation of a hypothesis but cannot be used to test a hypothesis because of limitation in their design. Also, because correlation studies refer to whole populations and not individuals, it is not possible to link exposure to occurrence of disease in the same person. This is a major limitation of ecologic studies.
- **Case reports and case series:** the most basic types of descriptive studies of individuals, they consist of detailed identification and reporting on a single subject (for case reports) or group of subjects (for case series). These are not considered true epidemiologic investigations.
- **Cross-section studies:** survey in which the status of an individual with respect to the presence or absence of both exposure and disease is assessed at the *same point in time*. Because exposure and disease are assessed at the same point in time, cross-section surveys cannot always indicate whether the exposure preceded the development of disease, or vice versa.

16. **A population study shows that, in parts of Ireland, Catholic districts have a significantly higher rate of suicide than Protestant districts. What type of descriptive study is this? What can be determined from an epidemiologic standpoint?**
This is an example of an ecologic study or, in other words, a population correlation study. It is the weakest of all epidemiologic surveys. Because ecologic studies compare groups rather than individuals, caution is required in drawing conclusions and identifying associations. The hazard in interpreting studies of this kind is labeled the *ecologic fallacy*.

17. **Explain the ecologic fallacy.**
It is an error in inference that occurs when an observed association is assumed to exist on an individual level. For instance, the high number of suicides in the Catholic districts may be caused by Protestants who live in those districts and commit suicide. However, ecologic studies can be useful in some ways because they are quick and easy, use existing data, and can help in formulating a hypothesis on which further investigation can be done.

18. **What is analytic epidemiology?**
Analytic epidemiology is the process of testing a specific hypothesis about a potential exposure and an outcome of interest. A study is performed to examine the relationship between the exposure to a risk factor and the outcome, typically a disease.

19. **List the types of analytic studies.**
Observational and experimental.

20. **Name the types of observational studies.**
Case-control and cohort studies. A case-control study may also be nested within a particular cohort study, in which case it is termed a *nested* case-control study.

KEY POINTS: PRINCIPLES OF EPIDEMIOLOGY

1. Epidemiology is the study of the distribution and determinates in the human population. It is the basic science and fundamental practice of public health.

2. The types of epidemiologic studies include ecologic, case study and case series, cross-section, cohort, and case-control.

3. The effect of differential age distribution in two comparable populations needs to be considered. By thus adjusting the rates, one attempts to compare the disease rates across population groups or to assess changes in rates over time. There are two central methods of rate adjustments: direct and indirect.

4. The standardized mortality ratio (SMR) may control for time-specific mortality by indirect standardization.

5. In calculating SMR, the age-specific rates from a standard population (e.g., county, state, or country) are multiplied by the person-years at risk in the study population (e.g., industry employees) to give the expected number of deaths. The observed number of deaths divided by the expected number, multiplied by 100, is the SMR.

21. **What are experimental studies?**
Experimental studies consist of clinical trials and are observed under predetermined conditions. In an experimental study, subjects are allocated into groups, which are given different exposures (typically treatment regimens) controlled by the researcher. To avoid bias, the groups being compared should be as similar as possible in all characteristics except the exposure. Randomization is a technique used to minimize bias.

22. **What is a case-control study?**
An epidemiologic study in which one compares the exposure among cases (i.e., individuals with disease) and controls (i.e., individuals without disease). A case-control study involves a group of persons with disease and a "matched" group, which is similar in all respects except for disease. A retrospective evaluation is conducted to determine who was exposed and who was not exposed.

23. **What is a cohort study?**
A study in which an exposed group and an unexposed group are followed over time to determine who develops the disease of interest. A cohort study provides the most direct evaluation of health and disease patterns in a population.

24. **What are the advantages and disadvantages of major epidemiologic study types?**
    See Table 2-1.

25. **List and explain the major methodologic issues that need to be considered in an epidemiologic study.**
    - **Precision**: reduction in random error, indicated by the variance of a measurement and associated confidence interval
    - **Validity**: reduction of systematic error or systematic bias, indicated by comparing what the study estimated and what it intended to estimate
    - **Selection bias**: any bias due to the manner in which participants were selected
    - **Information bias**: bias related to instruments and techniques used to collect information about exposure, health outcomes, or other factors
    - **Confounding bias**: caused by failure to account for the risk of other factors related to the exposure and health outcome. A confounder must be a risk factor for the disease, must be associated with the exposure, and must not be an intermediate step in the causal pathway between exposure and disease outcome

    Bowler RM, Cone JE: Occupational Medicine Secrets. Philadelphia, Hanley & Belfus, 1999.

TABLE 2-1.   ADVANTAGES AND DISADVANTAGES OF MAJOR TYPES OF EPIDEMIOLOGIC STUDIES

Study Design	Advantages	Disadvantages
Ecologic study	Quick and easy; acceptable for developing hypothesis for further studies.	Ecologic fallacy (see question 10). Does not look at individuals.
Case study/case series	Inexpensive and easy; good for very rare occurrences. Lays groundwork for future, more powerful studies.	Not a true epidemiologic study.
Cross-section study	Inexpensive, relatively quick, and easy. Good if population is difficult to access or define.	Selection bias: it may find survivor population with ill individuals gone. Measures prevalence only.
Cohort study	Measures risk.	Expensive Long follow-up period needed; individuals may be lost to follow-up. Large number of subjects required.
Case-control study	Less expensive and requires shorter time periods; good for rare diseases.	Recall bias: people with disease may tend to remember exposure better than controls.

Adapted from Bowler RM, Cone JE: Occupational Medicine Secrets. Philadelphia, Hanley & Belfus, 1999.

26. What is a rate?

The number of times a given event occurs over a specified time period, divided by the population at risk during that period. For convenience, rates are often given per 1000, 10,000, or 100,000 population at risk.

27. How are the main measures of mortality calculated?

The basic measures of disease in a population are mortality rates and morbidity rates. The following provides examples of the more common rates and how they are calculated.

$$\text{Crude death rate} = \frac{\text{No. of deaths in a year (all causes)}}{\text{Total population}} \times 1000$$

(for example, U.S. in 1977 = 8.8/1000 population)

$$\text{Cause-specific death rate} = \frac{\text{No. of deaths from specific causes}}{\text{Total population}} \times 100,000$$

(for example, cancer in U.S. in 1977 = 178.7/100,000 population)

$$\text{Age-specific death rate} = \frac{\text{No. of deaths among persons of specific age group in year}}{\text{Population in specified age group}} \times 100,000$$

(for example, cancer in age group 1–14 years = 4.9/100,000)

$$\text{Infant mortality rate} = \frac{\text{No. of deaths among children younger than 1 year of age in year}}{\text{No. of births in year}} \times 1000$$

From Principles of Epidemiology, 2nd ed. Atlanta, U.S. Department of Health and Human Services, Public Health Service, Centers for Disease Control and Prevention, Epidemiology Program Office, Public Health Practice Program Office, 1992.

28. Name some of the other rates describing morbidity and mortality.

Tables 2-2 and 2-3 illustrate several of the rates for examining the health characteristics of a population.

29. What is incidence?

Incidence is the number of new cases of a given disease at a specified time divided by the population at risk for that disease at that time.

30. What is prevalence?

Prevalence is the number of existing cases of a given disease at a specified time divided by the population at risk for that disease at that given time.

31. How are incidence and prevalence related?

A useful formula for estimating the prevalence of a given condition is

$$\text{Prevalence} = \text{incidence} \times \text{average duration of condition}$$

This formula is useful for estimation only and is more accurate as the average duration of the condition increases, as occurs in chronic diseases.

TABLE 2-2.   FREQUENTLY USED MEASURES OF MORBIDITY

Measure	Numerator (x)	Denominator (y)	Expressed per No. at Risk (10^n)
Incidence rate	No. of new cases of a specified disease reported during a given time interval	Average population during the same time interval	Varies: 10^n where n = 2, 3, 4, 5, 6
Attack rate	No. of new cases of a specified disease reported during an epidemic period	Population at start of the epidemic period	Varies: 10^n where n = 2, 3, 4, 5, 6
Secondary attack rate	No. of new cases of specified disease among contacts of known cases	Size of contact population at risk	Varies: 10^n where n = 2, 3, 4, 5, 6
Point prevalence	No. of current cases, new and old, of a specified disease at a given point in time	Estimated population at the same point in time	Varies: 10^n where n = 2, 3, 4, 5, 6
Period prevalence	No. of current cases, new and old, of a specified disease identified over a given time interval	Estimated population at mid-interval	Varies: 10^n where n = 2, 3, 4, 5, 6

From Principles of Epidemiology, 2nd ed. Atlanta, U.S. Department of Health and Human Services, Public Health Service, Centers for Disease Control and Prevention, Epidemiology Program Office, Public Health Practice Program Office, 1992.

TABLE 2-3. OTHER MEASURES OF MORTALITY

Measure	Numerator (x)	Denominator (y)	Expressed per No. at Risk (10^n)
Proportional mortality	No. of deaths assigned to a specific cause during a given time interval	Total no. of deaths from all causes during the same time interval	100 or 1000
Death-to-case ratio	No. of deaths assigned to a specific disease during a given time interval	No. of new cases of that disease reported during the same time interval	100
Neonatal mortality rate	No. of deaths under age 28 days during a given time interval	No. of live births during the same time interval	1000
Postneonatal mortality rate	No. of deaths from ages 28 days to, but not including, 1 year during a given time interval	No. of live births during the same time interval	1000
Maternal mortality rate	No. of deaths assigned to pregnancy-related causes during a given time interval	No. of live births during the same time interval	100,000

Adapted from Principles of Epidemiology, 2nd ed. Atlanta, U.S. Department of Health and Human Services, Public Health Service, Centers for Disease Control and Prevention, Epidemiology Program Office, Public Health Practice Program Office, 1992.

32. What are vital statistics?

Vital statistics are statistics enumerating births, deaths, fetal deaths, marriages, and divorces. The registration of these events is legally mandated; individual states are responsible for collecting the information and forwarding it to the National Center for Health Statistics.

33. What are some problems with gathering data from death certificates?

The only complete registry for all causes is for deaths, and the cause of death assignment on death certificates is often inaccurate. In addition, with a disease for which the case-to-fatality ratio is low (i.e., a disease unlikely to result in death when it occurs), the death rate is a gross underestimate of the incidence of the condition in the community. An example of this is non-melanoma skin cancer.

34. What is the main problem with morbidity reporting?

Morbidity reports, even when legally mandated, as is the case for certain infectious diseases (e.g., tuberculosis and sexually transmitted diseases), often results in severe underreporting.

35. What are crude rates?

Crude rates are rates that apply to an entire population, without taking into account any characteristics of the individuals within the population (e.g., age). To make meaningful comparisons between populations, rates must be adjusted.

36. What is meant by adjustment of rates?

The effect of differential age distribution in two comparable populations needs to be considered. By thus adjusting the rates, one attempts to compare the disease rates across population groups or to assess changes in rates over time. There are two central methods of rate adjustments: direct and indirect.

37. What is the direct method for rate adjustment?

The direct method applies observed age-specific rates to a standard population. This method is appropriate when each of the populations being compared is large enough to yield stable age specific rates. For example, the direct method is used for comparison of cancer rates over time. Crude mortality rates show a dramatic increase in cancer over the past few decades and would seem to provide strong evidence of a cancer epidemic. One must ascertain, however, to what extent the aging of the country's population has contributed to the apparent epidemic, and to what extent other factors, such as an increase in cancer-causing agents in the environment, might be responsible.

Table 2-4 shows an example of a calculation of a direct standardization of fictitious crude death rates.

LaDou J: Occupational and Environmental Medicine. 2nd ed. Stamford, CT: Appleton & Lange, 1997.

38. What is the indirect method of rate adjustment?

The indirect method applies the age-specific rates of a standard population to the age distribution of an observed population. To remove the variable effect of age by using the direct method of adjustment, a standard population is chosen. The number of people in each age group of the standard population is then multiplied by the appropriate age-specific rate in each of the study populations. This process generates the number of deaths one would expect in each age group; the sum is divided by the total standard population; the result is then multiplied by 100,000. Table 2-5 shows an example of a calculation of an indirect standardization of fictitious crude death rates.

39. When is it more useful to use the indirect method of standardization?

When the group being studied is relatively small, and thus likely to have unstable age-specific rates, it is more appropriate to use the indirect method over the direct method of standardization.

TABLE 2-4. DIRECT STANDARDIZATION OF CRUDE DEATH RATES OF TWO POPULATIONS, USING THE AVERAGED WEIGHTS AS THE STANDARD POPULATION (FICTITIOUS DATA)

Part 1 Calculation of the crude death rates

Age Group	Population Size		Population A Age-Specific Death Rate		Expected Number of Deaths	Population Size		Population B Age-Specific Death Rate		Expected Number of Deaths
Young	1000	×	0.001	=	1	4000	×	0.002	=	8
Middle-aged	5000	×	0.010	=	50	5000	×	0.020	=	100
Older	4000	×	0.100	=	400	1000	×	0.200	=	200
Total	10,000				451	10,000				308
Crude death rate			451/10,000 = 4.51%					308/10,000 = 3.08%		

Part 2 Direct standardization of the above crude death rates, with the two populations combined to form the standard weights

Age Group	Population Size		Population A Age-Specific Death Rate		Expected Number of Deaths	Population Size		Population B Age-Specific Death Rate		Expected Number of Deaths
Young	5000	×	0.001	=	5	5000	×	0.002	=	10
Middle-aged	10,000	×	0.010	=	100	10,000	×	0.020	=	200
Older	5000	×	0.100	=	500	5000	×	0.200	=	1000
Total	20,000				605	20,000				1,210
Standardized death rate			605/20,000 = 3.03%					1,210/20,000 = 6.05%		

From Jekel JF, Katz DL, Elmore JG: Epidemiology, Biostatistics, and Preventive Medicine, 2nd ed. Philadelphia, W.B. Saunders, 2001, p 33.

TABLE 2-5 INDIRECT STANDARDIZATION OF THE CRUDE DEATH RATE FOR MEN IN A COMPANY, USING THE AGE–SPECIFIC DEATH RATES FOR MEN IN A STANDARD POPULATION (FICTITIOUS DATA)

Part 1 Beginning data

Age Group	Men in the Standard Population				Men in the Company			
	Proportion of Standard Population		Age-Specific Death Rate	Observed Death Rate	Number of Workers		Age-Specific Death Rate	Observed Number of Deaths
Young	0.40	×	0.0001 =	0.00004	2000	×	? =	?
Middle-aged	0.30	×	0.0010 =	0.00030	3000	×	? =	?
Older	0.30	×	0.0100 =	0.00300	5000	×	? =	?
Total	1.00			0.00334	10,000			48
Observed death rate				0.00334, or 334/100,000				48/10,000, or 480/100,000

Part 2 Calculation of the expected death rate, using indirect standardization of the above rates and applying the age-specific death rates from the standard population to the number of workers in the company

Age Group	Men in the Standard Population				Men in the Company			
	Proportion of Standard Population		Age-Specific Death Rate	Observed Death Rate	Number of Workers		Standard Death Rate	Expected Number of Deaths
Young	0.40	×	0.0001 =	0.00004	2000	×	0.0001 =	0.2
Middle-aged	0.30	×	0.0010 =	0.00030	3000	×	0.0010 =	3.0
Older	0.30	×	0.0100 =	0.00300	5000	×	0.0100 =	50.0
Total	1.00			0.00334	10,000			53.2
Expected death rate								53.2/10,000, or 532/100,000

Continued

TABLE 2-5 INDIRECT STANDARDIZATION OF THE CRUDE DEATH RATE FOR MEN IN A COMPANY, USING THE AGE-SPECIFIC DEATH RATES FOR MEN IN A STANDARD POPULATION (FICTITIOUS DATA)—CONT'D

Part 3 Calculation of the standardized mortality ratio (SMR)

$$SMR = \frac{\text{Observed death rate for men in the company}}{\text{Expected death rate for men in the company}} \times 100$$

$$= \frac{0.00480}{0.00532} \times 100$$

$$= (0.90)(100) = 90$$

= Men in the company actually had a death rate that was only 90% of the value that would be expected, based on the death rates in the standard population.

From Jekel JF, Katz DL, Elmore JG: Epidemiology, Biostatistics, and Preventive Medicine, 2nd ed. Philadelphia, W.B. Saunders, 2001, p 34.

40. **When investigating cause-specific deaths in a cohort, which method of standardization is most likely used?**

The indirect method is most frequently used in cause-specific mortality in a cohort. The indirect method is frequently employed to compare the disease incidence or follow-up experience of a study group with that expected, as based on the experience of a larger population. With the indirect method, the age-specific rates for a standard population are multiplied by the person-years at risk in each group in the study series. The number of observed deaths is then compared with the number expected by means of a ratio.

41. **What is the standardized mortality ratio (SMR)?**

SMR is an example of indirect standardization. In calculating an SMR, the age-specific rates from a standard population (e.g., county, state, or country) are multiplied by the number of people at risk in the study population (e.g., industry employees) to give the expected number of deaths. The observed number of deaths divided by the expected number, multiplied by 100, is the SMR. An SMR may also control for time-specific mortality by indirect standardization.

WEBSITES

1. http://www.acepidemiology.org

2. http://www.apha.org/public_health/epidemiology.htm

BIBLIOGRAPHY

1. Bowler RM, Cone JE: Occupational Medicine Secrets. Philadelphia, Hanley & Belfus, 1999.

2. Doll R, Hill AB: The mortality of doctors in relation to their smoking habits: A preliminary report. Br Med J 1:1451–1455, 1954.

3. Hennekens CH: Epidemiology in Medicine. Boston, Little Brown & Company, 1987.

4. LaDou J: Occupational and Environmental Medicine, 2nd ed. Stamford, CT; Appleton & Lange, 1997.

5. Morris JN: Uses of Epidemiology, 3rd ed. Edinburgh, Churchill-Livingstone, 1975.

6. Wallace RB: Maxcy-Rosenau-Last's Public Health and Preventive Medicine, 14th ed. Stamford, CT, Appleton & Lange, 1998.

CHAPTER 3

MEASURING RISK

Mark Glover, BA, BM, BCh

NOTATION USED IN THIS CHAPTER

The observations in a controlled cohort study can be categorized as follows:

Risk factor present: **study** population
Risk factor absent: **control** population
Positive for outcome of interest: for instance, **disease**
Negative for outcome of interest: for instance, **no disease**

The table below is known as a 2×2 (two-by-two) table or a crossover table. This is a common method of summarizing research findings, in which the integer quantities represented by a, b, c, and d record the division of observations between each category.

	Study	Control
Disease	a	b
No disease	c	d

A total row can be added, as below, to simplify calculations:

	Study	Control
Disease	a	b
No disease	c	d
Total	a + c	b + d

Using this notation, we will see later that:

- Absolute risk in the study population (R_s) = a / (a + c)
- Absolute risk in the control population (R_c) = b / (b + d)
- Relative risk (RR) = R_s / R_c

1. **What is risk?**

   In everyday language, the word *risk* has many closely related meanings, which are often associated with bad outcomes. In statistical and epidemiologic terms, risk is simply an expression of probability. It is usually, but not invariably, the probability of an adverse event such as disease, injury, or death. Sometimes the nature of the risk depends on the perspective of the observer. For instance, there is a risk that you will lose money (an adverse event) if you buy a lottery ticket; but, if you do not win, the lottery organizers will profit (a beneficial event).

2. **What is absolute risk?**

   The absolute risk of an event is the probability of that event occurring. Only two pieces of information are required to calculate absolute risk, given by the equation

   $$\frac{\text{number of observations in which the occurrence of interest is found}}{\text{total number of observations}}$$

   If a denotes the total number of observations in which the occurrence of interest is found, and c denotes the total number of observations in which the occurrence of interest is *not* found, then the total number of observations is $a + c$, and the absolute risk of the occurrence of interest is expressed as

   $$\frac{a}{a + c}$$

3. **What values can an absolute risk take?**

   Because it is an expression of probability, a risk can have any value from 0–1. In some cases, risk can be given as a percentage with values from 0–100%. When the value is extremely small, risk can be expressed in occurrences of interest among a larger number of observations (for instance, 2.75 deaths per 100,000 population).

4. **What if it is not possible to collect every possible relevant observation?**

   It is seldom possible to include every possible relevant observation in a study. If a proportion of all possible observations is drawn randomly, however, and there are a observations in which the occurrence of interest is found and c observations in which the occurrence of interest is not found, the absolute risk may still be calculated from the fraction

   $$\frac{a}{a + c}$$

   So, as long as the observations that were taken are a proportionate representation of all possible relevant observations, the risk can be calculated correctly from a sample of the whole population.

5. **So information drawn from a sample of a given population is useful?**

   Very much so, as long as the sample is truly representative of the population that you are trying to characterize. For instance, assuming that in the United States there are 150,000 fatal and 450,000 nonfatal strokes annually, the risk of a stroke being fatal in the United States each year is

   $$150,000 / (150,000 + 450,000) = 150,000 / 600,000 = 0.25.$$

   If every thousandth stroke victim within the United States was selected randomly for a survey over a year, 600 cases would be collected for the study. If those cases were a proportionate representation of all stroke sufferers in the United States, 150 would die and 450 would survive. The risk of a stroke being fatal, calculated from the collected observations, is

   $$150 / (150 + 450) = 150 / 600 = 0.25$$

   This is the same risk as would be calculated from the whole population of stroke victims.

6. **What is the difference between a risk and a rate?**
    Naming conventions are not totally consistent throughout scientific literature, but, strictly speaking, a rate has a denominator with units that include time. For instance, 25 deaths per 100,000 population **per year**. A risk does not require time within the denominator; for instance, 2.6 deaths per 100 open-heart operations.

7. **What is the difference between an incidence risk and an incidence rate?**
    This is another epidemiologic convention that can cause confusion. Incidence is a measure of how many cases of interest develop within a population over time, typically 1 year. Incidence **risk** is an absolute risk, calculated by dividing the number of new cases developing in a year by the number of people who are disease-free at the beginning of the year. Incidence **rate** is an expression of the number of new cases developing in a year divided by the average number of people who are disease-free over the year.

8. **Give examples of how incidence risk and incidence rate are determined.**
    Let's take an extreme example of a population of 1000 with a serious disease that causes 720 of them to die in 1 year. The incidence **risk** of mortality in that population will be 720 / 1000 = 0.72 / year.
    The simplest way to work out the average number of the population who are disease-free over the year is to calculate the mean of those disease-free at the beginning (1000) and end of the year (1000 – 720 = 280). In this case, the average is (1000 + 280) / 2 = 1280 / 2 = 640. The incidence **rate** of mortality in that population is 720 / 640 = 1.125. Unlike a risk, incidence **rate** can, therefore, exceed 1 in some circumstances. An alternative way of describing the denominator for incidence **rate** is the mean time that one person will need to wait before contracting the disease.

9. **Do these differences have significant effect on study results?**
    The difference between calculated values for incidence risk and rate is minimal in the majority of cases. Two factors are responsible for this:
    - Most diseases affect quite small proportions of a population, and few will leave the group at risk.
    - The rate denominator often remains stable as new persons at risk replace those who leave the group. For instance, a population remains moderately stable if births roughly balance out deaths.

10. **What are high and low values for absolute risk?**
    There is no standard. A single value of absolute risk in isolation does not tell you whether it is high or low. The only way that this can be done using absolute risk is by comparing findings in two or more sets of observations.

11. **Give an example of how high and low values for absolute risk are determined. How did the risk of divorce in the United Kingdom compare with that in Greece in 2002?**
    Government statistics show that the risk of divorce in Greece in 2002 was 1.1 per 1000 population, while the risk of divorce in United Kingdom in 2002 was 2.7 per 1000 population. The risk of divorce was clearly greater in the United Kingdom than it was in Greece. The conclusion is straightforward in this case because such figures are usually derived from centrally kept national registers covering the whole population. If only a sample of each national population had been taken, statistical tests would have been required to establish that the differences in the risks were significant.

12. **How does comparative risk differ from absolute risk?**
    Absolute risk, when quoted in isolation, does not give any information about whether it is high or low. Also, it is not possible to calculate absolute risk from all study designs. In contrast,

measures of comparative risk allow us to produce single terms that compare the risk in different populations and, hence, give some idea of relative magnitude of risks. These measurements can be estimated from a wider range of studies. Methods commonly used to describe comparative risk are relative risk, odds ratio, and attributable risk.

13. What is the best method for measuring comparative risk?

No method gives a perfect description if quoted in isolation. Worse still, the figures can be used to give a highly distorted impression of the truth. As a result, two of the greatest challenges to health care professionals are interpreting the results correctly, and then explaining a specific risk to a layman in a manner that is both relevant to the individual and conveys its true magnitude. Different measures are best suited to specific uses.

14. With what do comparative risk measurements compare risk?

Risks in any two groups can be compared, but many research projects compare the observations of the one or more groups being studied with observations of a control group. The study groups have some unifying inherent or acquired characteristics, often termed *risk factors*. The control group is chosen from a group that lacks the risk factor. Through comparison, the effect upon risk of outcome can be assessed.

15. What form do risk factors take?

Risk factors take many forms, including inherited, environment, and lifestyle-related. Examples of risk factors include the following:

- Genetic defect, extreme of morphology, or extreme of physiologic measurement such as blood pressure
- Infective or environment exposures
- Exposure to therapeutic or toxic substances

16. What is relative risk?

Relative risk (RR), or risk ratio, is a measure of the absolute risk in one population as a proportion of the absolute risk in another. Usually, but not invariably, the higher risk is used for the numerator. Because the control group often has the lower risk, relative risk is usually expressed as

$$R_s/R_c$$

The relative risk measurement is favored by researchers looking for the strength of an association between a risk factor and an outcome of interest. In some cases, however, relative risk can mislead.

17. How can the use of relative risks be misleading?

Using the formula above, if there is a rare disease with an absolute risk of 1 in 10 million per year, and a food additive is found to increase the absolute risk to 5 in 10 million per year, then the relative risk for those who consume the food additive would be 5. If there is a more common but equally serious disease with an absolute risk of 1 in 10,000 per year and a pharmaceutical preparation is found to increase the absolute risk to 1.2 in 10,000 per year, the relative risk for those who take the pharmaceutical is 1.2. Learning that the food additive increases the risk of a disease fivefold and that the medicine increases the risk of a disease by a factor of 1.2 could lead to the conclusion that greater benefits are to be gained by avoiding the food additive.

18. The above example does not seem misleading. Why is it?

First, let us examine the benefit of removing the food additive since it showed a higher relative risk than the medication. This removal would lead to 4 fewer cases of disease in a population of 1 million. Despite its lower relative risk, however, avoiding the medication would lead to 20 fewer cases in a population of 1 million (1.2 cases in 10,000 − 1 case in 10,000 = 0.2 cases in 10,000 = 20 cases in 1 million). The difference in background risk between the two diseases can have a profound effect, and it is often best to calculate the actual anticipated change in terms of raw numbers of cases.

19. What are odds?
The probability of an event expressed as a proportion of the probability that it will not occur is known as the odds of an event. The probability of an event in a study population is R_s and, because the sum of all probabilities must equal 1, the probability that the event will not occur is $(1 - R_s)$. Odds are calculated by dividing the probability of the event by the probability that it will not occur. The odds of the event occurring in the study population can, therefore, be expressed in the form $R_s / (1 - R_s)$.

20. Give an example of how odds are used.
Each time an unbiased die is thrown, the probability of a score of 1 is 1 in 6 and the probability of the score being other than 1 is 5 in 6. The odds of a score of 1, therefore, is $\frac{1}{6} / \frac{5}{6} = \frac{1}{5} = 0.2$.

21. Define an odds ratio.
The odds ratio, or the cross-products ratio, is the odds of an occurrence of interest in the study population, expressed as a proportion of the odds of the same occurrence in a control population. This ratio can be expressed as

$$[R_s / (1 - R_s)] / [R_c / (1 - R_c)]$$

$$= [R_s \times (1 - R_c)] / [R_c \times (1 - R_s)]$$

22. This seems confusing. Is there an easier way to calculate the odds ratio?
Yes. Fortunately, the raw figures can also be used. Referring to the generic 2×2 table, the odds of a positive outcome in the study population would be a/c. The odds of a positive outcome in the control population would be b/d. Therefore, the odds ratio would be

$$(a/c) / (b/d)$$

$$= ad/bc$$

23. Why is it typically impossible to calculate relative risk from a case-control study?
A case-control study involves selection of one group with disease (or other outcome of interest) and one without. The number of individuals with the risk factor under investigation in each group is then determined. Remember, risk can be calculated from a sample only if it reflects the proportions in the whole population.

24. Is it ever possible to calculate relative risk from a case-control study?
It is possible to calculate the risks from a case-control study in only one of the following unlikely circumstances:
- If the study includes all possible members of the appropriate populations
- If the numbers of individuals in the sample groups with and without risk factors are present in the same proportions as the population from which they are drawn.

25. Why is the probability of having a risk factor in the presence or absence of disease seldom calculated from the results of a case-control study?
There is no more than a very loose relationship between the risk of disease in the presence or absence of a risk factor and the probability of having that risk factor in the presence or absence of the same disease. This information would be of academic interest only and of no predictive use at all.

26. Give an example of the above problem.
Small lungs with low forced vital capacities (FVCs) have been shown to be associated with pulmonary barotrauma (PBT) during pressurized submarine escape training ascents. Some

fictitious records of ascents at a submarine escape training facility are shown in the following table:

	Low FVC	FVC normal or larger	Total
PBT	39	83	122
No PBT	7547	240,168	247,715
Total	7586	240,251	247,837

Because the whole population is recorded, risks can be calculated. The risk of pulmonary baro-trauma with a low FVC is $^{39}/_{7586} = 5.1$ in 1000 ascents. The probability of a low FVC in the presence of pulmonary barotrauma is much greater at $^{39}/_{122} = 0.47$ and is clearly not a good measure of the risk of each ascent undertaken.

27. **What measure can be used to obtain clinically useful predictive information from a case-control study?**
    The odds ratio can be used to illustrate the strength of association between risk factor and out-come in both cohort and case-control studies. A mathematic property inherent within the odds ratio that makes it particularly useful for case-control studies is that the odds ratio does not require risk factors to be present in the same proportions as the population from which the sam-ples were drawn. In addition, the odds ratio possesses symmetry such that

    $$\frac{\text{odds of disease with a risk factor present}}{\text{odds of disease when a risk factor is absent}}$$

    is equal to

    $$\frac{\text{odds of a risk factor in those with disease}}{\text{odds of a risk factor in those without disease}}$$

    As a result, the odds ratio gives a consistent and meaningful measure of the relationship between risk factor and disease, whichever way it is calculated. Also, if the outcome of interest occurs only rarely, the odds ratio is very close to the relative risk.

28. **Give a worked illustration of the symmetry of odds ratios.**
    For this example, we will use the generic 2×2 table at the beginning of the chapter. We saw ear-lier that the odds ratio of disease in the presence of a risk factor is given by $(a/c) / (b/d) = ad/bc$. Re-titling the generic 2×2 table to represent the findings of a case-control study, in which the numbers were divided between outcome and risk factor in the same proportions as before, gives us the following:

	Risk factor present	Risk factor absent
Study group (formerly Disease)	a	b
Control group (formerly No disease)	c	d

The odds of a risk factor in the presence of disease equals a/b. The odds of a risk factor in the absence of disease equals c/d. The odds ratio is a/b / c/d= ad/bc, the same as the odds ratio cal-culated using odds of disease.

29. **Give an illustration of the circumstances required for odds ratio to closely approximate to relative risk.**

    The relative risk in a cohort study is given by the expression R_c/R_s. In terms of raw numbers from the generic 2×2 table, relative risk is equal to $[a/(a + c)]/[b/(b + d)]$. As the outcome of interest becomes rarer, both a and b tend to zero and the relative risk tends to

    $$[a/(0 + c)]/[b /(0 + d)]$$
    $$= (a/c) / (b/d)$$
    $$= ad/bc,$$

    which is the same as the odds ratio. So if a disease is rare, the odds ratio is a close estimate of the relative risk.

30. **Apply the odds ratio to the example of the submarine escape training tank.**

    The results from the submarine escape training tank are repeated below:

	Low FVC	FVC normal or larger	Total
PBT	39	83	122
No PBT	7547	240,168	247,715
Total	7586	240,251	247,837

    The risk of PBT with a low FVC (R_s) is $a / (a + c) = 39 / 7586 = 5.1$ in 1000
    The risk of PBT with FVC normal or larger (R_c) is $b / (b + d) = 83 / 240{,}251$
    $$= 3.5 \text{ in } 10{,}000$$
    The relative risk (RR) is $R_s / R_c = 5.1 \times 10^{-3} / 3.5 \times 10^{-4} = 14.9$
    The odds of PBT with a low FVC is $a / c = 39 / 7547 = 5.2 \times 10^{-3}$
    The odds of PBT with FVC normal or larger is $b / d = 83 / 240{,}168 = 3.5 \times 10^{-4}$
    This gives an odds ratio of $(5.2 \times 10^{-3}) / (3.5 \times 10^{-4}) = 15$
    The odds of a low FVC with PBT is $a / b = 39 / 83 = 0.47$
    The odds of a low FVC without PBT is $c / d = 7547 / 240{,}168 = 0.031$
    This gives an odds ratio of $0.47 / 0.031 = 15$

    Note the odds ratio is identical calculated either way. Also note that the odds ratio and relative risk are very similar because clinically apparent PBT is rare.

31. **How do relative risk and odds ratio differ?**

    From the answers above, we can see that relative risk can be calculated from a cohort study but not from a case-control study, whereas an odds ratio can be calculated from either type of study. The odds ratio closely approximates the relative risk when the outcome of interest is rare and the groups are representative of the populations from which they are drawn. Neither relative risk nor odds ratio gives any clue to the magnitude of risk in the background population or control group.

32. **What is the importance of the denominator when assessing risk?**

    Care must be taken to define and fully understand the denominator, as it could have a significant impact on the interpretation of results. Similarly, it is important to ensure that any risks used for comparison have the appropriate denominators to allow that comparison. There is little point, for instance, in making an uncorrected or unqualified comparison between a risk measured over 2 years with another risk measured over 3 years. The population from which observations may be taken embraces a wide range of possibilities.

33. **Can there really be that many choices for a denominator?**

    Yes. For instance, consider the question, "What is the risk of fatality as a result of a road traffic accident in the United States?" The denominator could be any of the following figures:
    - Individuals in the United States

- Individuals involved in road traffic accidents in the United States
- Journeys made
- Minutes spent in a car
- Miles driven

All would be acceptable, but the answers will be very different. An appreciation of this fact is particularly important in comparing the risk with another activity, such as parachuting, in which there are fewer deaths overall but the total number of individuals exposed, duration of exposure, and distance traveled are all much smaller.

34. Give an example of how different denominators affect calculation of risk.

The following fictitious figures relate to mortality while SCUBA diving and level of training in a diving association:

- There are 60,000 active members in the diving association.
- At any one time, 12,000 of the association's divers are initial trainees.
- The average duration of a dive for a trainee is 20 minutes.
- A trainee will typically be required to complete 20 dives in 1 year to gain full qualification.
- Once qualified, members dive, on average, 10 times each year.
- The average duration of a dive for a qualified member is 40 minutes.
- There are 24 fatalities while diving each year, 25% (6) of which involve trainees.

So are trainees at greater risk of a fatal incident?

If we take numbers of individuals per year as the denominator, $6/12,000 = 5$ in 10,000 trainees having a fatal accident each year and $1/48,000 = 3.75$ in 10,000, qualified members will have a fatal accident each year. The conclusion would be that trainees are at greater risk.

If we analyze by numbers of dives per year, $6/(12,000 \times 20) = 2.5$ in 100,000 trainee dives result in a fatal incident and $18/(48,000 \times 10) = 3.75$ in 100,000 dives by qualified members result in a fatal incident. The conclusion in this case would be that qualified members were at greater risk.

If we look at numbers of minutes of diving per year, $6/(12,000 \times 20 \times 20) = 1.25$ fatalities in 1 million trainee dive minutes and $18/(48,000 \times 10 \times 40) = 0.9375$ fatalities in 1,000,000 dive minutes by qualified members. The conclusion here would be that trainees are at greater risk.

If cumulative risk of diving fatality is used, each diver will have been a trainee, and then additional risk would be accrued while continuing to dive as a qualified member. The conclusion here would be that members qualified for the longest period were at greater risk.

There is clearly a requirement for common sense to be applied in deciding on an appropriate denominator, and the example above shows how difficult it can be to demonstrate precisely what is required.

35. What is attributable risk?

Attributable risk is the risk in the study group less the risk in the control group. It can be calculated from the equation

$$R_s - R_c$$

This is the most appropriate measure of change in risk when making a decision for an individual, such as whether the risk of side effects from taking a drug is tolerable or not.

36. Give an example of attributable risk.

If a study finds that the risks of dying in middle age are 0.4 and 0.22 for a smoker and a non-smoker, respectively, then the attributable risk for smoking is $0.4 - 0.22 = 0.18$.

37. What is the attributable risk percent?

This is the attributable risk expressed as a percentage of the absolute risk in the study group, which can be calculated from the formula:

$$\frac{100\% \times (R_s - R_c)}{R_s}$$

The formula gives the proportion of cases of the disease under investigation in the exposed population for which a risk factor is responsible.

38. Give an example of attributable risk percent.
In the smoker study from question 36, the attributable risk percent is $(100\% \times 0.18) / 0.4 = 45\%$.

39. How do relative risk and attributable risk differ?
Relative risk gives no information on the actual change in risk magnituder, whereas attributable risk does. Relative risk, therefore, has limited use when making decisions for an individual. The two are related by the formula

$$\text{Attributable risk} = R_c \times (\text{relative risk} - 1)$$

As stated earlier, relative risk is most commonly used for assessing the strength of association between risk factor and outcome. The approximate value of relative risk can be estimated from a case-control study, whereas attributable risk cannot. In addition, relative risk is often a better indicator of the interaction between different risk factors. The interaction is usually seen as a relatively constant multiplier, to be applied to the relative risk for each individual risk factor.

40. Give an example of how relative and attributable risks differ in their sensitivity to absolute magnitude of risk.
If R_s is 0.075 and R_c is 0.05, then attributable risk is $0.075 - 0.05 = 0.025$ and relative risk is $0.075 / 0.05 = 1.5$.

If R_s is 0.75 and R_c is 0.5, then attributable risk is $0.75 - 0.5 = 0.25$ but, despite the tenfold increase in overall risk, relative risk is unchanged at $0.75 / 0.5 = 1.5$.

41. What is the population attributable risk?
Population attributable risk predicts the reduction in risk achievable if a risk factor is removed from a population. It is calculated by multiplying attributable risk by prevalence of exposure to the risk factor, and can be expressed by the formula

$$(R_s - R_c) \times \text{proportion of population exposed}$$

The population attributable proportion is a measure of what proportion of a disease in a population is attributable to the risk factor. This can be expressed by the formula

$$\frac{(R_s - R_c) \times \text{proportion of population exposed}}{(R_s \times \text{proportion of population exposed}) + [R_c \times (1 - \text{proportion of population exposed})]}$$

Since relative risk $(RR) = R_s/R_c$, the population attributable proportion can be written in terms of RR as follows:

$$\frac{\text{proportion of population exposed} \times (RR\text{-}1)}{1 + [\text{proportion of population exposed} \times (RR\text{-}1)]}$$

Therefore, in the right circumstances, an odds ratio can be used to estimate population attributable proportion. The proportion can be expressed as the population attributable percent, given by multiplying the formula by 100%, as follows:

$$\frac{100\% \times (R_s - R_c) \times \text{proportion of population exposed}}{(R_s \times \text{proportion of population exposed}) + [R_c \times (1 - \text{proportion of population exposed})]}$$

This can also be calculated in terms of relative risk:

$$\frac{100\% \times [\text{proportion of population exposed} \times (RR - 1)]}{1 + [\text{proportion of population exposed} \times (RR - 1)]}$$

All of these measures are used to compare the effects of possible public health strategies.

42. Give an example of population attributable proportion.

Consider a fictitious cohort study of risk of decompression illness (DCI), taken in 1 year, with 500 divers with a variation in heart anatomy known as a patent foramen ovale (PFO) controlled against 500 divers without a PFO. The results are summarized as follows:

	PFO	Control
DCI	2	1
No DCI	498	499
Total	500	500

It is widely believed that a PFO, or any other right-to-left circulatory shunt, increases the risk of DCI. Some 30% of individuals within the general population have a PFO, and some surveys have shown that a similar proportion of divers have a PFO.

In this study, the absolute risk of DCI with a PFO is 2/500 = 0.004 and the absolute risk of DCI in an individual with no PFO is 1/500 = 0.002. The relative risk is 0.004/0.002 = 2 and the odds ratio is 2/0.998 = 2.

- The attributable risk is 0.004 − 0.002 = 0.002
- The attributable risk percent is 0.002/0.004 = 50%
- The population attributable risk is 0.002 × 0.3 = 0.0006
- The population attributable proportion is 0.0006/[(0.004 × 0.3) + (0.002 × 0.7)] = 0.0006/(0.0012 + 0.0014) = 0.0006/0.0026 = 0.23.

The population attributable percent, therefore, will be 23%. So, according to these results, routine closure of PFOs in divers would reduce the overall risk of DCI by 23% in this population.

KEY POINTS: MEASURING RISK

1. Absolute risk is probability of an event such as illness, injury, or death.

2. An absolute risk gives no indication of how its magnitude compares with others'.

3. The odds ratio closely approximates the relative risk if the disease is rare.

4. The odds ratio and the relative risk are used to assess the strength of association between risk factor and outcome.

5. The attributable risk is used to make risk-based decisions for individuals.

6. Population attributable risk measures are used to inform public health decisions.

43. What if the control group differs from the study group in ways (other than the risk factor under investigation) that might influence the outcome of interest?

It is not unusual for characteristics, such as age and sex, to influence outcome, independent of the risk factor being studied. In studies of cardiovascular mortality, for instance, fewer would be expected to die in a younger population with a greater proportion of females. In such cases, the odds ratios might need to be modified to account for differences in samples.

44. What techniques can be used to make the odds ratio more representative?

One technique is stratum matching, in which the same number of cases and controls are drawn from each age/sex group. Another technique is to calculate the odds ratio for each group and then summate them.

45. **How do you calculate the odds ratio in a case-control study with matched controls?**

In case-control studies, age/sex matched controls are often selected for each case. Sometimes more than one matched control is selected for each case to enhance statistical significance. The resulting information can be tabulated in the following format:

		Controls	
		Risk factor present	Risk factor absent
Cases	Risk factor present	a	b
	Risk factor absent	c	d

In this case, the odds ratio is calculated from b/c. If you want to understand why this should be so, read a large reference book and then let me know, too!

WEBSITES

1. http://www.amstat.org/sections/epi/SIE_Home.htm

2. http://www.biostat.ucsf.edu/epidem/epidem.html

BIBLIOGRAPHY

1. Bland M: An Introduction to Medical Statistics. New York, Oxford University Press, 1995.

2. Daly LE, Bourke GJ: Interpretation and Uses of Medical Statistics, 5th ed. Oxford, Blackwell Science Ltd., 2000.

3. Gigerenzer G: Calculated Risks: How to Know When Numbers Deceive You. New York, Simon & Schuster, 2002.

4. Kirkwood BR: Essentials of Medical Statistics. Oxford, Blackwell Science Ltd., 1988.

CHAPTER 4

DATA SOURCES AND SURVEILLANCE

Michael D. Lappi, DO, PhD

1. **What is a survey?**
    A method of monitoring behaviors associated with disease, attributes that affect disease risk, knowledge or attitudes that influence health behaviors, the use of health services, and self-reported disease occurrence. In general, surveys are relatively inexpensive and provide a reliable and reproducible method for gathering information from any number of individuals.

2. **Name some of the weaknesses of surveys.**
    First, surveys do not employ the scientific method in their design or implementation. In addition, surveys are typically a cross-section instrument for gathering information, meaning that data about both exposure and outcome are gathered at the same time. In cross-section surveys, it is impossible to ascertain any information about the temporal relationship between a potential risk factor and an outcome. Bias can also be a major problem in the collection and interpretation of survey data.

3. **What types of diseases do surveys tend to identify?**
    Surveys tend to identify both chronic and less severe diseases, for the simple reason that people are more likely to be present and healthy enough to answer question, compared with people suffering from severe, rapidly progressive diseases.

4. **What are some examples of surveys?**
    One example of a common survey is the cross-section survey, through which a diverse population may be studied at a single point in time. Examples of well-known surveys include a census, which studies a large population, and a poll, which focuses on political objectives.

5. **Explain surveillance.**
    Surveillance is the systematic collection, analysis, and dissemination of disease data pertaining to groups of people, and is designed to detect early signs of disease. Surveillance is performed at many levels for a large variety of populations and is a cornerstone of preventive medicine.

6. **Give the primary purpose of medical surveillance.**
    To prevent disease and injury and, ultimately, to improve quality of life.

7. **What are the types of surveillance?**
    One way to describe surveillance systems is to categorize them as either active or passive.

8. **Describe active surveillance.**
    Active surveillance requires dedicated efforts of personnel and, typically, frequent management of collection sources to identify cases. Because of the required levels of effort, active surveillance is done on a select topic for a limited amount of time. Active surveillance is much more expensive than passive surveillance.

9. **Provide are some examples of active surveillance.**
    Two examples are the ongoing Framingham Heart Study and the Nurses' Health Study.

10. **Describe passive surveillance.**

   In contrast to active surveillance, passive surveillance relies on timely and thorough reporting of disease to the appropriate agencies. Passive surveillance is far more commonly employed and holds the expectation that requested information will be supplied as directed by the physician, clinic staff, medical center, laboratory, or other responsible party.

KEY POINTS: SURVEYS AND SURVEILLANCE

1. Surveys are an effective way of gathering information, although they do not employ the scientific method.

2. Surveys are more likely to capture information about chronic or less severe disease processes.

3. The goal of surveillance is to prevent disease and injury.

4. Surveillance is a cornerstone of public health practice.

5. Baseline rates are made possible by surveillance data.

11. **What is the most widely used example of passive surveillance?**

   The most common example of passive surveillance is the collection of reportable diseases by local, state, and federal agencies, and the tabulation of that data by the Centers for Disease Control and Prevention (CDC), published in the Morbidity and Mortality Weekly Report.

12. **Define baseline rate.**

   A baseline rate consists of data, typically presented as incidence rates over time, that describe previous patterns of the studied disease process to establish typical occurrences under the necessary parameters. Examples of the topics studied through baseline rates may range from issues as simple as the number of sick days taken by a group of co-workers over the course of the past 5 years to issues such as the number of cancer cases in this same group over a 5-year period.

13. **What information must we consider when examining baseline data and trends?**

   The reported data may well be indicative of a change in the incidence of a particular outcome. However, one must always consider whether there has been a change in the way the outcome is defined, detected, or reported over the period in question.

14. **How are baseline rates useful?**

   They set the standard to which all future occurrences of a given topic (e.g., sick days or cancer) may be compared with detect atypical events. This fact underlies the importance of surveillance: without baseline data, there would be no standard for comparison.

15. **What are secular trends?**

   These are occurrences of health outcomes of interest over time, typically years. Figure 4-1 illustrates both a trend in the number of cases of acquired immunodeficiency syndrome (AIDS) between 1984 and 1993, and also the effect of changing case definition. If it were not known that the case definition for AIDS was changed in 1993, one might mistakenly assume an acute change in the baseline (i.e., expected number of cases).

16. **What are vital statistics?**

   They are critical events in the lifespan of an individual. In the United States, these events are birth, death, marriage, divorce, and fetal death. These data are initially gathered at the local level

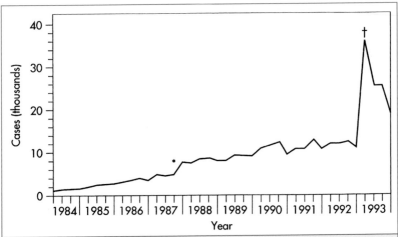

Figure 4-1. AIDS cases by quarter year reported in the United States, 1984–1993. *In October 1987 the case definition and diagnostic criteria were revised. †In 1993 the case definition was revised again. (From CDC: Update: Trends in AIDS diagnosis and reporting under the expanded surveillance definition for adolescents and adults—United States, 1993. MMWR 43[32]:826-828, 1994.)

and forwarded to the state. At the state level, this information is summarized, and then the report is sent to the National Center for Health Statistics (NCHS).

17. **Explain the purpose of the National Center for Health Statistics (NCHS). What data does it collect?**

The NCHS is the branch of the CDC designated as the focal point in the collection of vital statistics within the United States. Information contained in birth and death certificates from the states, number and characteristics of births and deaths, and marriages and divorces are all tracked by the NCHS. The collection of these data is considered to be a national responsibility; data are eventually submitted to the United Nations.

18. **What is the U.S. census? What are its characteristics?**

The U.S. census is a federal program established in 1790 to characterize and quantify the population of the states, mostly for taxation and military service. The first census asked only six questions: name of the head of the household; number of persons living in the household; number of free white males, 16 years old or older, living in the household; number of free white males under the age of 16 living in the household; and the sex and color of all of the other persons living in the household.

19. **How often is the U.S. census performed?**

This constitutionally mandated process is begun every April 1 of years ending in zero, and the results are typically reported within 1 to 2 years. While the census offers a reasonable assessment of the demographics of the population, the validity of the results is directly based on the quality of the data submitted.

20. **What information is gathered during the census? From whom?**

Census information is gathered from every U.S. household, as identified by an extensive computer cross-referencing network, incorporating census data, government address lists, and U.S.

Postal Service address systems. In addition, census workers physically identify living quarters not recognized by this process through door-to-door census data collection.

There are two versions of the census: a short form and a longer, more detailed form. In general, one in every six households will receive the longer version. If the census is not filled out and sent back by the required date, then a census worker will pay that household a visit. The worker will verbally ask the head of the household the questions and will fill in the appropriate answers on a printed form. The long-form questionnaire for the 2000 census is shown in Table 4-1.

TABLE 4-1. LONG FORM OF THE 2000 U.S. CENSUS	
Population	**Housing**
Ancestry	Farm residence
Disability	Heating fuel
Grandparents as caregivers	Number of rooms and number of bedrooms
Income in 1999	Plumbing and kitchen facilities
Labor force status	Telephone service
Language spoken at home and ability to speak English	Units in structure
Marital status	Utilities, mortgage, taxes, insurance, and fuel costs
Migration (residence in 1995)	Value of home or monthly rent paid
Occupation, industry, and class of worker	Vehicles available
Place of birth, citizenship, and year of entry	Year moved into residence
Place of work and journey to work	Year structure built
School enrollment and educational attainment	
Veteran status	
Work status in 1999	

21. **Identify potential shortfalls in the census system.**
Issues regarding the validity of the census focus on geographic irregularity and question variability. Because of the almost constant fluctuation in growth characteristics in a given area, the census cannot use standard geographic boundaries or base results according to zip code. Similarly, census questionnaires are tailored to address areas relevant to the administration of the current government and, therefore, are not directly comparable from census to census.

22. **What is the current population of the United States based on the 2000 census?**
As of the 2000 census, the population of the United States is 281,421,906, representing a 13.2% increase (i.e., a growth of 32,712,033) in population over the previous results, reported in 1990.

23. **Describe the primary reportable disease network administered by the CDC.**
The National Notifiable Disease Surveillance System (NNDSS) is responsible for the collection of data from physicians, hospitals, clinics, and laboratories. The system is designed to track data from the reporting site to the local and state health departments and, finally, to the CDC in Atlanta, Georgia.

24. **What are the reportable diseases, as defined by the CDC, within the United States in 2005?**
See Table 4-2.

TABLE 4-2.

AIDS

Anthrax

Arboviral neuroinvasive and
nonneuroinvasive diseases

- California serogroup virus disease
- Eastern equine encephalitis virus
  disease
- Powassan virus disease
- St. Louis encephalitis virus disease
- West Nile virus disease
- Western equine encephalitis virus
  disease

Botulism

- Botulism, foodborne
- Botulism, infant
- Botulism, other (wound and
  unspecified)

Brucellosis

Chancroid

Chlamydia trachomatis, genital infections

Cholera

Coccidioidomycosis

Cryptosporidiosis

Cyclosporiasis

Diphtheria

Ehrlichiosis

- Ehrlichiosis, human granulocytic
- Ehrlichiosis, human monocytic
- Ehrlichiosis, human, other, or
  unspecified agent

Enterohemorrhagic *Escherichia coli*

- Enterohemorrhagic *Escherichia
  coli,* O157:H7
- Enterohemorrhagic *Escherichia
  coli,* shiga toxin positive, serogroup
  non-O157
- Enterohemorrhagic *Escherichia
  coli,* shiga toxin positive (not
  serogrouped)

Giardiasis

Gonorrhea

Haemophilus influenzae, invasive disease

Hansen disease (leprosy)

Hantavirus pulmonary syndrome

Hemolytic uremic syndrome,
postdiarrheal

Hepatitis, viral, acute

- Hepatitis A, acute
- Hepatitis B, acute
- Hepatitis B virus, perinatal infection

Hepatitis, viral, chronic

- Chronic Hepatitis B
- Hepatitis C virus infection (past or
  present)

Human immunodeficiency virus (HIV)
infection

- HIV infection, adult (≥13 years)
- HIV infection, pediatric (<13 years)

Influenza-associated pediatric mortality

Legionellosis

Listeriosis

Lyme disease

Malaria

Measles

Meningococcal disease

Mumps

Pertussis

Plague

Poliomyelitis, paralytic

Psittacosis

Q fever

Rabies

- Rabies, animal
- Rabies, human

Rocky Mountain spotted fever

Rubella

Rubella, congenital syndrome

Salmonellosis

Severe Acute Respiratory Syndrome-
associated Coronavirus (SARS-CoV)
disease

Shigellosis

Smallpox

TABLE 4-2.—CONT'D

Streptococcal disease, invasive, group A	Syphilis, congenital
Streptococcal toxic-shock syndrome	▪ Syphilitic stillbirth
Streptococcus pneumoniae, drug-resistant, invasive disease	Tetanus
	Toxic-shock syndrome
Streptococcus pneumoniae, invasive, in children <5 years	Trichinellosis (Trichinosis)
	Tuberculosis
Syphilis	Tularemia
▪ Syphilis, primary	Typhoid fever
▪ Syphilis, secondary	Vancomycin–intermediate *Staphylococcus aureus* (VISA)
▪ Syphilis, latent	
▪ Syphilis, early latent	Vancomycin–resistant *Staphylococcus aureus* (VRSA)
▪ Syphilis, late latent	
▪ Syphilis, latent unknown duration	Varicella (morbidity)
▪ Neurosyphilis	Varicella (deaths only)
▪ Syphilis, late, nonneurological	Yellow fever

25. **What is the purpose of the National Center for Injury Prevention and Control (NCIPC) section of the CDC?**
It works to reduce morbidity, disability, mortality, and costs associated with injuries.

26. **List the five major concerns of the NCICP.**
- Child maltreatment
- Intimate partner violence
- Sexual violence
- Suicide
- Youth violence

27. **The National Center for Health Statistics (NCHS) is responsible for which surveys?**
- National Health and Nutrition Examination Survey (NHANES): collects data on chronic disease prevalence and conditions (including undiagnosed conditions), risk factors, diet and nutrition status, immunization status, infectious disease prevalence, health insurance, and measures of environment exposures.
- National Health Care Survey (NHCS): obtains information about the facilities that supply health care, the services rendered, and the characteristics of the patients served.
- National Health Interview Study (NHIS): annual nationwide survey of about 36,000 households in the United States; a principal source of information on the health of the civilian noninstitutionalized population.
- National Immunization Survey (NIS): list-assisted, random-digit dialing telephone survey which began data collection in April 1994 to monitor child immunization.
- National Survey of Family Growth (NSFG): the main purpose of the 1973–1995 surveys was to provide reliable national data about marriage, divorce, contraception, infertility, and the health of women and infants in the United States.
- State and Local Area Integrated Telephone Survey (SLAITS): supplements current national data collection strategies by providing in-depth state and local data to meet various program and policy needs in our ever-changing health care system.

28. **How does the NCHS use the information that they obtain in these surveys?**
As described by NCHS, these statistics allow them to do the following:
- Document the health status of the population and of important subgroups
- Identify disparities in health status and use of health care by race and ethnicity, socioeconomic status, region, and other population characteristics

- Describe experiences with the health care system
- Monitor trends in health status and health care delivery
- Identify health problems
- Support biomedical and health services research
- Provide information for making changes in public policies and programs
- Evaluate the impact of health policies and programs

29. **What is the world's largest telephone survey?**

The Behavioral Risk Factor Surveillance System (BRFSS), which tracks health risks in the United States. The BRFSS questionnaire is designed by a group of state coordinators and CDC staff.

30. **What are the parts of the BRFSS survey?**

Currently, the questionnaire has three parts: (1) the core component, consisting of the fixed core, rotating core, and emerging core; (2) optional modules; and (3) state-added questions. All health departments must ask the core component questions without modification in wording; however, the modules are optional.

31. **Describe the core component of the BRFSS.**

The fixed core is a standard set of questions asked by all states. It includes queries about current behaviors that affect health (e.g., tobacco and alcohol use, physical activity, seeking of preventive medicine care) and questions on demographic characteristics. The rotating core is made up of two distinct sets of questions, each asked in alternating years by all states, addressing different topics.

32. **Can the optional portions of the survey be modified by the states?**

No. Optional CDC modules are sets of questions on specific topics (e.g., smokeless tobacco) that states elect to use on their questionnaires. Although the modules are optional, CDC standards require that, if they are used, they must be used without modification. Module topics have included survey items on smokeless tobacco, oral health, cardiovascular disease, and firearms.

33. **What is the purpose of a disease registry?**

A disease registry is designed to focus on a specific condition or disease to track reportable characteristics for further analysis and research. Typical diseases tracked in registries include cancer and congenital birth defects. The Occupational Lung Disease Registry and the Occupational Disease Registry catalog and follow diseases associated with the workplace.

34. **Are registries used only to track diseases?**

No. In fact, twin registries are used in an effort to delineate between environment and genetic causes of different diseases, as well as overall health and wellness.

35. **What is the purpose of the Agency for Toxic Substances and Disease Registry (ATSDR)?**

The ATSDR acts as the lead public health agency for implementing the health-related provisions of the Superfund (the Comprehensive Environmental Response, Compensation, and Liability Act of 1980). ATSDR is charged with assessing health hazards at specific hazardous waste sites, helping to prevent or reduce exposure and the illnesses that result, and increasing knowledge and understanding of the health effects that may result from exposure to hazardous substances.

36. **Who controls the data collected from federal programs such as Medicare and Medicaid?**

The Centers for Medicare & Medicaid Services (CMS) is a federal agency within the U.S. Department of Health and Human Services dedicated to the operation of select federal programs. Programs for which CMS is responsible include Medicare, Medicaid, the State Children's Health Insurance Program (SCHIP), the Health Insurance Portability and Accountability Act of 1996 (HIPAA), and the Clinical Laboratory Improvement Amendments (CLIA).

The Medicare Current Beneficiary Survey (MCBS), an example of a survey within CMS, is the only comprehensive source of health characteristics for the entire spectrum of Medicare beneficiaries.

37. **Who controls medical data obtained by the U.S. military and the Veterans Administration? What information do they collect?**
The Defense Medical Surveillance System (DMSS) is the central repository of medical surveillance data for the U.S. Armed Forces. Data in the DMSS document statuses of and changes in demographic and military characteristics (e.g., service, rank, and military occupation) of all service members. In addition, they document significant military (e.g., assignments and major deployments) and medical (e.g., ambulatory clinic visits, hospitalizations, immunizations, and deaths) experiences of service members throughout their military careers.

The DMSS receives data from multiple sources and integrates them in a continuously expanding relational database. Longitudinal records are established and constantly updated for all individuals who have served in the Armed Forces since 1990. Categories of special interest are major deployments, pre- and post-deployment health assessments, hospitalizations (in fixed military medical facilities), and ambulatory visits (to fixed military medical facilities). The DMSS also maintains of a central repository for serologic specimens.

38. **What is the Bureau of Labor Statistics?**
Under the U.S. Department of Labor, the Bureau of Labor Statistics is the principal fact-finding agency for the Federal Government in the broad field of labor economics and statistics. It provides an outstanding amount of information on all aspects of the U.S. labor force, including topics such as inflation, wages, productivity, health, demographics, and unemployment.

39. **What branch of the U.S. Department of Labor focuses on worker safety?**
The Occupational Safety and Health Administration (OSHA). Their mission is to assure the safety and health of America's workers by setting and enforcing standards; providing training, outreach, and education; establishing partnerships; and encouraging continual improvement in workplace safety and health.

40. **Name the federal agency responsible for conducting research and making recommendations for the prevention of work-related injury and illness.**
The National Institute for Occupational Safety and Health (NIOSH). It is part of the CDC Department of Heath and Human Services and has no enforcement powers.

41. **Break down the number and rate of occupational deaths in the United States by sex, race, and age group.**
See Table 4-3.

TABLE 4-3. NUMBER AND RATE* OF TRAUMATIC OCCUPATIONAL DEATHS, BY SEX, RACE, AND AGE GROUP—UNITED STATES, 1980–1997

Characteristic	No.	(%)	Rate
Sex			
Male	97,053	(93)	8.6
Female	6886	(7)	0.8
Unknown	6	(<1)	—
Race			
White	88,392	(85)	5.0
Black	11,478	(11)	5.6
Other	3167	(3)	4.8
Unknown	908	(1)	—
Age group (yrs)			
16–17	969	(1)	2.1
18–19	2714	(3)	3.8
20–24	10,791	(10)	4.5
25–34	26,390	(25)	4.7
35–44	22,881	(22)	4.5
45–54	18,213	(18)	5.2
55–64	14,108	(14)	6.9
≥65	7779	(7)	13.3
Unknown	100	(<1)	—
Total	**103,945**	**(100)**	**5.1**

*Per 100,000 workers. Rates not calculated for "unknown" or "not classified" categories.

42. Compare the number of fatal work injuries in the United States for the years 1992–2003.
    See Figure 4-2.

43. Which industries historically have the highest number of occupationally related deaths?
    - Construction (19,179 deaths, or 19% of reported deaths)
    - Transportation, communications, and public utilities (17,489, or 17% of reported deaths)
    - Manufacturing (15,490, or 15% of reported deaths)

44. Which industries historically have the highest occupational death rates?
    - Mining (30 deaths per 100,00 workers)
    - Agriculture, forestry, and fishing (19 deaths per 100,000 workers)
    - Construction (15 deaths per 100,000 workers)

45. Which industries had the highest number of occupationally related deaths in 2003?
    - Construction (1126 deaths)
    - Transportation and warehousing (805 deaths)
    - Agriculture, forestry, fishing, and hunting (707 deaths)

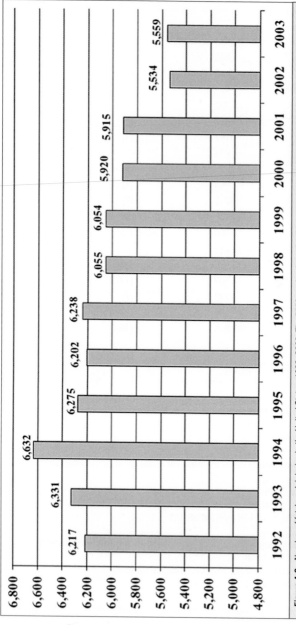

Figure 4-2. Number of fatal work injuries in the United States, 1992–2003. The 5559 work-related fatalities recorded in 2003 represent a small increase from the revised total reported for 2002. Data from 2001 excludes fatalities from September 11 terrorist attacks. (Source: U.S. Department of Labor, Bureau of Labor Statistics, Census of Fatal Occupational Injuries, 2003.)

46. **Which industries had the highest rates of occupationally related deaths in 2003?**
   - Agriculture, forestry, fishing, and hunting (31.2 deaths per 100,000 workers)
   - Mining (26.9 deaths per 100,000 workers)
   - Transportation and warehousing (17.5 deaths per 100,000 workers)
     Figure 4-3 summarizes the number and rate of fatal occupational injuries by industry sector in 2003.

47. **Which states historically have the highest numbers and rates of occupational fatalities?**
   The greatest number of fatal occupational injuries have occurred in California (10,712 deaths, or 10% of total U.S. fatal occupational injuries), Texas (10,294, or 10%), Florida (6269, or 6%), Illinois (4582, or 4%), and Pennsylvania (4402, or 4%). Fatal occupational injury rates have been highest in Alaska (22.7 per 100,000 workers), Wyoming (15.8 per 100,000), Montana (11.8 per 100,000), Idaho (10.4 per 100,000), and West Virginia (10.1 per 100,000).

48. **Which states had the highest number of occupational fatalities in 2002?**
   In 2002, the greatest number of fatal occupational injuries occurred in California (478 deaths), Texas (417 deaths), Florida (354 deaths), Ohio (202 deaths), Georgia (197 deaths), Illinois (190 deaths), and Pennsylvania (188 deaths). (See Table 4-4.)

49. **Which worker vital characteristics account for the majority of occupational deaths in the United States from 1992–2002?**
   Although the races, genders, ages, and employment status of these workers certainly comprise an all-encompassing list, the majority of occupational fatalities in the United States from 1992–2003 were white male wage and salary workers between the ages of 25 and 34 years (*see* Table 4-5).

50. **What information is available regarding worldwide health initiatives?**
   The World Health Organization (WHO) provides a wide range of useful information regarding numerous health programs throughout the globe. This data is best accessed by using either the World Health Organization Library Service (WHOLIS) or the World Health Organization Statistical Information Service (WHOSIS).

51. **Name the library data system that contains WHO publications.**
   WHOLIS is the WHO library database available on the web. WHOLIS indexes all WHO publications from 1948 onwards and articles from WHO-produced journals and technical documents from 1985 to the present. An on-site card catalogue provides access to the pre-1986 technical documents.

52. **Name the electronic database system that contains World Health Organization epidemiologic and statistic information.**
   WHOSIS is a guide to epidemiologic and statistic information at WHO. Most WHO technical programs develop health-related epidemiologic and statistic information, which they make available on the WHO website.

53. **What type of information can be found on WHOSIS?**
   Information available includes
   - Burden of disease statistics
   - WHO mortality database
   - Statistic annexes of the World Health Report
   - Statistics by disease or condition
   - Heath personnel
   - External sources for health-related statistic information

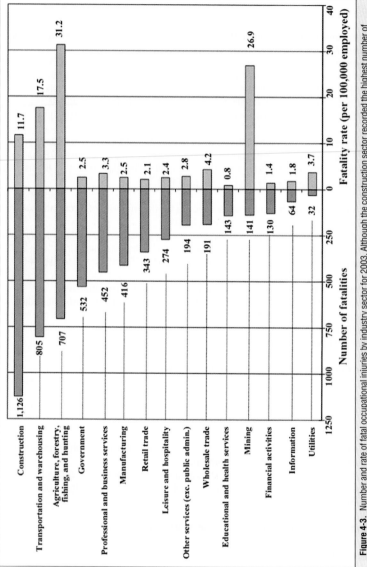

Figure 4-3. Number and rate of fatal occupational injuries by industry sector for 2003. Although the construction sector recorded the highest number of fatal work injuries, the highest fatality rates were in agriculture, forestry, fishing, and hunting. (Source: http://www.bls.gov/iif/oshwc/cfoi/cfch0002.pdf)

TABLE 4-4. OCCUPATIONAL FATALITIES BY STATE OF INCIDENT

Characteristics	1992	1993	1994	1995	1996	1997	1998	1999	2000	2001	2002
Total	6217	6331	6632	6275	6202	6238	6055	6054	5920	5915	5534
State of Incident											
Alabama	145	138	153	150	155	139	135	123	103	138	102
Alaska	91	66	60	78	63	51	43	42	53	64	42
Arizona	67	55	79	86	77	61	74	70	118	87	101
Arkansas	82	71	85	92	88	102	86	76	106	68	80
California	644	657	639	646	641	651	626	602	553	515	478
Colorado	103	99	120	112	90	120	77	106	117	139	123
Connecticut	42	31	35	32	35	32	57	38	55	41	39
Delaware	11	13	15	12	18	17	11	14	13	10	11
District of Columbia .	8	25	21	16	19	23	13	14	13	11	8
Florida	329	345	358	391	333	366	384	345	329	368	354
Georgia	204	230	249	237	213	242	202	229	195	237	197
Hawaii	28	26	21	24	27	19	12	32	20	41	24
Idaho	45	43	50	53	62	56	51	43	35	45	39
Illinois	250	252	247	250	262	240	216	208	206	231	190
Indiana	148	136	195	156	143	190	155	171	159	152	136
Iowa	110	88	74	54	70	80	68	80	71	62	57
Kansas	82	99	106	95	85	93	98	87	85	94	89
Kentucky	117	143	158	140	141	143	117	120	132	105	146
Louisiana	153	171	187	139	134	137	159	141	143	117	103
Maine	19	20	22	18	23	19	26	32	26	23	30
Maryland	103	82	80	86	82	82	78	82	84	64	102

Continued

TABLE 4-4 OCCUPATIONAL FATALITIES BY STATE OF INCIDENT—CONT'D

Characteristics	1992	1993	1994	1995	1996	1997	1998	1999	2000	2001	2002
Massachusetts	67	85	74	66	62	69	44	83	70	54	46
Michigan	143	160	180	149	155	174	179	182	156	175	152
Minnesota	103	113	82	84	92	72	88	72	68	76	81
Mississippi	123	121	126	128	103	104	113	128	125	111	94
Missouri	140	131	155	125	140	123	145	165	148	145	175
Montana	65	38	50	34	50	56	58	49	42	58	51
Nebraska	43	78	83	54	56	46	56	66	59	57	83
Nevada	49	38	41	51	52	55	60	58	51	40	47
New Hampshire	10	13	14	12	11	23	23	14	13	9	19
New Jersey	138	145	114	118	100	101	103	104	115	129	129
New Mexico	35	55	54	58	60	50	48	39	35	59	63
New York (except N.Y.C.)	127	154	180	158	169	155	149	121	122	120	140
New York City	187	191	184	144	148	109	94	120	111	100	100
North Carolina	169	214	226	187	191	210	228	222	234	203	169
North Dakota	20	30	21	28	23	35	24	22	34	25	25
Ohio	203	190	209	186	201	201	186	222	207	209	202
Oklahoma	78	86	97	200	87	104	75	99	82	115	92
Oregon	88	84	80	73	85	84	72	69	52	44	63
Pennsylvania	242	241	354	233	282	259	235	221	199	225	188
Rhode Island	17	16	12	11	6	11	12	11	7	17	8
South Carolina	100	87	83	115	109	131	111	139	115	91	107

Characteristics	1992	1993	1994	1995	1996	1997	1998	1999	2000	2001	2002
South Dakota	28	28	31	26	32	23	28	46	35	35	36
Tennessee	145	154	170	179	152	168	150	154	160	136	140
Texas	536	529	497	475	514	459	523	468	572	536	417
Utah	59	66	66	51	64	66	67	54	61	65	52
Vermont	11	7	8	16	7	9	16	14	15	6	11
Virginia	175	135	164	132	153	166	177	154	148	146	142
Washington	97	112	118	109	128	112	113	88	75	102	86
West Virginia	77	66	61	56	66	53	57	57	46	63	40
Wisconsin	135	138	109	117	108	114	97	105	107	110	91
Wyoming	26	36	35	32	28	29	33	32	36	40	33

Source: Bureau of Labor Statistics, 2003.

TABLE 4-5. WORKER VITAL CHARACTERISTICS

Characteristics	1992	1993	1994	1995	1996	1997	1998	1999	2000	2001	2002
Employee status											
Wage and salary workers	4975	5025	5370	5074	4977	4970	4804	4904	4736	4781	4481
Self-employed	1242	1303	1262	1201	1225	1268	1251	1150	1184	1134	1053
Sex											
Men	5774	5842	6104	5736	5688	5761	5569	5612	5471	5442	5092
Women	443	489	528	539	514	477	486	442	449	473	442
Age											
Under 16 years	27	29	25	26	27	21	33	26	29	20	16
16 – 17 years	41	39	42	42	43	41	32	46	44	33	25
18 – 19 years	107	102	114	130	125	113	137	122	127	122	92
20 – 24 years	544	508	545	486	444	503	421	451	446	441	436
25 – 34 years	1556	1521	1567	1409	1362	1325	1238	1175	1163	1142	1023
35 – 44 years	1538	1584	1619	1571	1586	1524	1525	1510	1473	1478	1403
45 – 54 years	1167	1204	1310	1256	1242	1302	1279	1333	1313	1368	1253
55 – 64 years	767	811	866	827	855	875	836	816	831	775	784
≥ 65 years	467	522	525	515	504	520	541	565	488	530	495

Characteristics	1992	1993	1994	1995	1996	1997	1998	1999	2000	2001	2002
Race or ethnic origin											
White	4711	4665	4954	4599	4586	4576	4478	4410	4244	4175	3926
Black or African American	618	649	695	684	615	661	583	616	575	565	491
Hispanic or Latino	533	634	624	619	638	658	707	730	815	895	841
American Indian or Alaskan Native	36	46	39	27	35	34	28	54	33	48	40
Asian, Native Hawaiian or .... Pacific Islander	192	206	211	188	188	218	164	180	185	182	140
Multiple races	—	—	—	—	—	—	—	—	—	6	4
Other races or not reported	127	131	109	158	140	91	95	63	68	44	92

Source: Bureau of Labor Statistics, 2003.

WEBSITES

1. http://www.bls.gov/iif/oshwc/cfoi/cfch0002.pdf

2. http://www.bls.gov/iif/oshwc/cfoi/cftb0186.pdf

BIBLIOGRAPHY

1. Jekel JF, Katz DL, Elmore JG: Epidemiology, Biostatistics, and Preventive Medicine. Philadelphia, W.B. Saunders, 2001, pp 20–39.

2. Rom WM (ed): Environmental and Occupational Medicine, 3rd ed. Philadelphia, Lippincott-Raven, 1998, pp 19–25.

3. Rothman KJ, Greenland S: Modern Epidemiology. Philadelphia, Lippincott Williams & Wilkins, 1998, pp 435–447.

4. Wallace RB (ed): Maxcy-Rosenau-Last's Public Health and Preventive Medicine, 14th ed. Stamford, CT, Appleton & Lange, 1998.

CHAPTER 5

DISEASE TRANSMISSION AND OUTBREAK INVESTIGATION

Thomas H. Winters, MD and Ann M. Zaia, NP-C, MSN, MHA

GENERAL CONCEPTS

1. **What are the components of the epidemiologic triangle?**
   Host, agent, and environment. A host is the living organism capable of becoming infected, an agent is a factor that must be present (or potentially missing) for the occurrence of a disease, and an environment is an extrinsic force or situation affecting the host's opportunity to be exposed to the agent. A vector may be present to bring the agent to the host (Fig. 5-1).

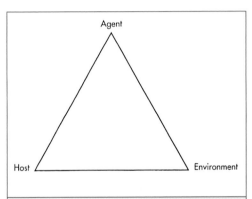

Figure 5-1. Epidemiologic triangle model of causation. (From Principles of Epidemiology, 2nd ed. Atlanta, U.S. Department of Health and Human Services, Public Health Service, Centers for Disease Control and Prevention, Epidemiology Program Office, Public Health Practice Program Office, 1992.)

2. **Explain the relationship among the legs of the epidemiologic triangle.**
   Well-known as one of the elemental ecologic models in public health, the epidemiologic triangle is often used to explain the concept of disease causation. The host, agent, and environment are the necessary components of the triangle. When viewed as an equilateral triangle, any change in one leg will inevitably alter one or both of the remaining legs, causing either an increase or decrease in the frequency of the disease state.

3. **List some of the characteristics affecting disease frequency for the three components of the epidemiologic triangle.**
   Host characteristics
   - Age
   - Genetics
   - Sex
   - Socioeconomic status
   - Immunity

Agent characteristics
- Environment stability
- Virulence
- Resistance

- Infectivity
- Pathogenicity

Environment characteristics
- Biologic (e.g., vectors and reservoirs)
- Physical (e.g., heat and population density)
- Social (e.g., culture)

4. **What is the only known reservoir for the measles virus?**

   The site where an infectious disease survives is considered a reservoir. While reservoirs can include both animate organisms and inanimate matter, humans are the only known reservoir for the measles virus.

5. **Explain how infectious agents are transmitted, and describe direct and indirect transmission.**

   Disease transmission is classified as either direct or indirect. Direct transmission entails the transfer of the infectious agent by physical contact with lesions, blood, saliva, or other secretion. Infectious transfer from a direct aerosolization, such as a sneeze in another person's face, is also typically considered direct. Indirect transmission occurs when the infectious agent spends a variable intermediate period within or upon some substance or living organism prior to causing disease in the host.

6. **By which mechanisms can direct and indirect transmission take place?**

   Direct transmission implies close contact, which is typically described as being within three feet of the infected individual in the case of droplet spread (e.g., coughing, sneezing, and talking). Activities that can cause immediate transfer of an infectious agent into a susceptible portal of entry, such as kissing, biting, or sexual intercourse, are methods of direct transmission. Indirect transmission, on the other hand, is either vehicle- or vector-borne. A vehicle may be any inanimate object or biologic material (e.g., blood and tissue) that acts as an intermediary in transferring the infective agent to the host.

7. **Is hepatitis A acquired through direct or indirect transmission?**

   Hepatitis A is acquired via the fecal-oral route, which is considered indirect transmission. Pathogens must be capable of withstanding the environment outside their natural host for some period of time to be a viable source of indirect transmission.

   An example of this type of transmission might occur when an employee (i.e., reservoir) with hepatitis A, working in a local fast-food restaurant, fails to wash his hands after using the bathroom. The employee then returns to the food preparation station and makes your deluxe jumbo burger. In the process, fecal material infected with hepatitis A is transferred to your lunch. Famished as usual, you consume every bite. In about a month you notice the onset of flu-like symptoms and yellow sclera. Your astute powers of self-diagnosis reveal that you have hepatitis A. Because you never actually came into direct contact with the person who prepared your burger, you acquired the hepatitis A via indirect transmission.

   In contrast, direct transmission could occur when your best friend, who is nursing a cold, shows his less considerate side and sneezes in your face. So remember: to help prevent both direct and indirect transmission, always cover your mouth when you cough and wash your hands afterward!

8. **What is the chain of infection?**

   The chain of infection is the mechanism by which transmission of an agent occurs from its reservoir to its host. Figure 5-2 is a useful schematic illustrating the chain of infection.

9. **How are infectivity, pathogenicity, and virulence different?**

   According to the Centers for Disease Control and Prevention (CDC), infectivity is the proportion of persons exposed to a causative agent who develop an infectious disease. Infectivity can be measured by secondary attack rate. Pathogenicity is the ability of an organism to cause a disease state (morbidity), whereas virulence is the ability to actually cause death (mortality). The

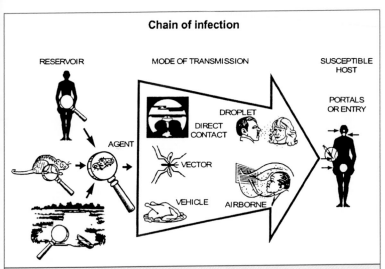

Figure 5-2. Chain of infection. (From Principles of Epidemiology, 2nd ed. Atlanta, U.S. Department of Health and Human Services, Public Health Service, Centers for Disease Control and Prevention, Epidemiology Program Office, Public Health Practice Program Office, 1992.)

virulence of a pathogen can be altered. For example, the discovery of penicillin in the late 1930s significantly reduced the mortality rate of pneumococcal bacteremia from about 90% to 10%.

10. **What percentage of hospital-acquired bacteria infections is resistant to at least one of the antibiotics most frequently prescribed for their treatment?**

    The degree to which a disease-causing microorganism does not respond to drugs intended to eradicate it is known as its resistance. Overprescription of antibiotics has led to the mutation of many bacteria as a survival mechanism against our labors to eliminate them. This sophisticated strategy on the part of the bacteria has led to either the reduction or, in some cases, the complete ineffectiveness of current treatment regimens. More than 70% of hospital-acquired bacteria infections may demonstrate some level of resistance to at least one drug commonly used to treat them. At the level of the host, multiple factors determine resistance, including sex, age, socioeconomic status, baseline health, and nutrition status. In addition, genetic make-up determines individual resistance to various diseases (termed *innate resistance*).

11. **The concept of apparent and inapparent infection was conceived by which recipient of the 1928 Nobel Prize in Medicine?**

    Dr. Charles Jules Henry Nicolle was the winner. While conducting research on guinea pigs he had infected with typhus, Nicolle made a rather astonishing discovery: some of the infected guinea pigs, despite displaying no apparent typhus symptoms, were capable of spreading the disease. Today we more commonly term *apparent* and *inapparent* infections as *symptomatic* or *asymptomatic* infections.

12. **Name the two types of immunity.**

    - Passive immunity: antibodies formed in another person or animal are transferred to an individual. This type of immunity is short-lived.
    - Active immunity: antigens are transferred to an individual via a portal of entry. Once the antigen enters the body, it stimulates the immune system to produce antibodies. Initial exposure of an antigen and the subsequent host antibody formation are termed the primary response. Immunoglobulin M (IgM) is the main antibody produced during the primary

immune response, whereas immunoglobulin G (IgG) dominates at the time of reexposure, when cellular memory kicks in. The formation of IgG explains why active immunity is more persistent than passive immunity.

13. **What types of immunity can be acquired artificially?**
Both passive and active immunity may be acquired by either natural or artificial means.

KEY POINTS: DISEASE TRANSMISSION

1. Host, agent, and environment make up the epidemiologic triangle.

2. Infectious agents can be transmitted directly or indirectly.

3. Pathogenicity is the ability to cause diseases, whereas virulence is the ability to cause death.

4. The primary attack rate is the number of people who become ill divided by all those at risk.

5. Both passive and active immunity can be acquired through natural or artificial means.

6. An epidemic is a greater than expected frequency of a disease or illness for a given population and time period.

---

14. **Acquired immunity may be conferred in one of two ways: either artificially or naturally. Name the method employed in providing an individual with artificially acquired immunity.**
Administration of a prophylactic vaccine such as measles-mumps-rubella (MMR), inactivated poliomyelitis, or pneumococcal pneumonia confers artificially acquired immunity by exposing an individual to the antigens of a particular viral or bacterial pathogen.

15. **An emergency department physician from a local hospital arrives at your practice, stating that he was just stuck with a needle from a known hepatitis B-positive patient. He is concerned because he never received the hepatitis B vaccine (he was "too busy" to get it). As part of the standard blood borne pathogens protocol in your practice, you immediately administer hepatitis B immune globulin, based on your understanding that it will confer what type of immunity?**
Passive artificially acquired immunity. Hepatitis B immunoglobulin is indicated for acute exposures to hepatitis B surface antigen (HBsAg) in an individual who has either never received the hepatitis B vaccine or is a known nonresponder to the vaccine. This temporary form of immunity promotes development of anti-hepatitis B surface antibodies in approximately 1–6 days, with a duration of protection from 2–6 months. Best when administered within 24 hours, it should be given no later than 7 days after the exposure to be effective. In the case of the previously unvaccinated doctor, or a patient whose titer has fallen below a protective level, the hepatitis B vaccine series should be given at the same time that hepatitis immunoglobulin is administered (at separate sites) to confer active, artificially acquired, long-term immunity.

16. **The initial fluid secreted by the mammary glands after childbirth is known as colostrum. You encourage new mothers to breast-feed because you are aware that colostrum provides which type of immunity to the infant?**
Colostrum provides naturally acquired passive immunity. This occurs when antibodies contained in the colostrum are ingested by the infant, cross the intestinal mucosa, and are transported to the blood.

17. **What is herd immunity?**
Herd immunity is the immunity of a group or community (Fig. 5-3). In other words, it is the resistance of a group to invasion and spread of an infectious agent based on the resistance of a high proportion of members of that group. This includes a vaccinated group.

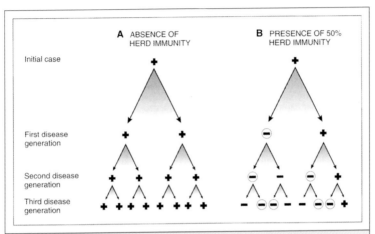

Figure 5-3. The effect of herd immunity on the spread of infection. The diagrams illustrate how an infectious disease such as measles can spread in a susceptible population if each infected person were exposed to two other persons. In the absence of herd immunity (A), the number of cases doubles in each disease generation. In the presence of 50% herd immunity (B), the number of cases remains constant. The plus sign represents an infected person, the minus sign represents an uninfected person, and the circled minus sign represents an immune person who will not pass the infection to others. (From Jekel JF, Katz DL, Elmore JG: Epidemiology, Biostatistics, and Preventive Medicine, 2nd ed. Philadelphia, W.B. Saunders, 2001.)

18. **Why is the loss of herd immunity against smallpox in the United States an increasing public health concern in relationship to biologic warfare?**
Since the World Health Organization officially declared smallpox to be eradicated worldwide in 1980, with the last naturally occurring case in 1977, immunization programs for this disease have ceased. Without the benefit of naturally occurring disease or active artificial immunity in the form of vaccination, herd immunity cannot develop. Therefore, should smallpox be released as a weapon of bioterrorism, the lack of group immunity may make it a deadly threat.

19. **What change at the molecular level effects a change in antigenicity of the human immunodeficiency virus (HIV), making it difficult to develop an effective HIV vaccine?**
A process known as antigenic drift is the culprit. Antigenic drift is the development of point mutations over time. In certain viruses, like HIV, this can happen quite easily because of a high replication rate. Antigenic drift causes small changes in the virus, which decrease the host immune response by lowering the efficacy of the cellular memory of T and B cells.

20. **Is antigenic drift the same thing as antigenic shift?**
No. Antigenic shift is a major and more immediate change than antigenic drift in the surface proteins of a virus, leading to extensive alteration in genetic information. The influenza virus is notorious for its tendency toward antigenic drift and antigenic shift, resulting in many historically significant epidemics.

21. **As the newly appointed physician for a local public health department, your first charge is to investigate a repeating pattern of cases of aseptic meningitis in the community. Because you aced your epidemiology class in medical school, you recall that the proper epidemiologic terminology for this excess pattern would also be what?**

    Periodicity. Figure 5-4 shows the pattern of aseptic meningitis in the United States from 1986–1994.

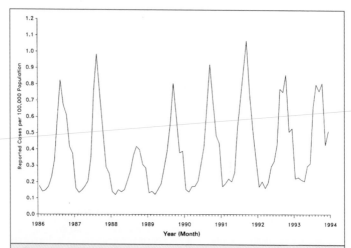

Figure 5-4. Aseptic meningitis, reported cases per 100,000 population by month, United States, 1986–1993. (From CDC: Summary of notifiable diseases, United States, 1993. MMWR 49:49, 1994.)

22. **You are paged in the middle of the night and notified that one of your patients, a 65-year-old woman with a history of congestive heart failure and chronic obstructive pulmonary disease, was just admitted to the hospital with a *Streptococcus pneumoniae* infection. The attending physician in the emergency department assures you that the patient has been started on penicillin and will be just fine. Comforted by his reassuring tone, you return to bed. The next afternoon you are paged by the nurse on the floor, who tells you that your patient had become septic and was transferred to the medical intensive care unit. What went wrong?**

    Antibiotic resistance. Penicillin-resistant *Streptococcus pneumoniae* was first documented in New Guinea in 1967, and later appeared in the United States in the 1980s.

    Bacterial resistance is a natural consequence of the evolutionary process and is achieved via the process of adaptation. While the antibiotic itself is not the actual cause of the resistance, the drug's efforts to eliminate the infection trigger the bacterium's survival instincts, which ultimately leads to genetic changes. Essentially, resistance occurs because the bacterium makes an end-run around our efforts to stop it by either natural resistance (i.e., vertical evolution via spontaneous mutation) or acquired resistance (i.e., horizontal evolution via the acquisition of genes for resistance from another organism through transduction, conjugation, or transformation).

    In the case of penicillin resistance, the bacteria reinvent themselves in an effort to survive and elicit enzymes that destroy the drug or alter its ability to bind to and damage the cell walls. While it is crucial that we employ every effort to slow this process down, the reality is that, because of rapid bacterial cell growth and the sophistication of genetic processes such as mutation and selection, it is unlikely we will ever be capable of stopping it.

23. **The increase in pneumococcal infections during winter months is best described by which epidemiologic term?**
Seasonal variation is the cyclic pattern for attack rates related to common pathogens. Particular pathogens are more likely to occur at certain times of the year. *Streptococcus pneumoniae*, *Staphylococcus aureus*, and influenza A and B are more likely to appear in the winter, legionellosis usually comes in the summer, and *Mycoplasma* species show up in summer and fall in the Northern Hemisphere. Figure 5-4 shows both the periodicity of aseptic meningitis and the seasonal variation of the illness.

24. **As the head of infectious disease in a small, rural hospital, staff often turn to you with exposure questions. You receive a call from the nurse manager of the emergency department, notifying you that a patient was just admitted with chickenpox pneumonia. She is concerned because one of her newly hired nurses, who had cared for this patient, was just notified by employee health that her varicella titer had come back negative. Based on our knowledge of the incubation period of varicella, what advice would you give the nurse manager?**
Health care workers are vigilant of chickenpox patients because of the long incubation period and the need to furlough the nonimmune workers (i.e., those with no natural immunity and those nonimmune workers who did not receive a live attenuated varicella virus vaccine) for 10–21 days after exposure. The incubation period is the time interval between initial contact with the infectious agent and the first appearance of symptoms associated with the varicella infection. The varicella virus has a long incubation period of 14–21 days. According to the Massachusetts Department of Public Health, susceptible health care workers shall be excluded from work from the 10th through 21st days after their last exposure. However, if the nurse in question receives varicella zoster immunoglobulin (VZIG), her exclusion should be extended to 28 days after exposure. Exclusion of workers is often emphasized 4 days before the beginning of the incubation period, because the varicella virus is communicable 2 days before onset of rash. Should the nurse contract the disease, she must remain out of work until she is no longer contagious, typically 6–8 days or until all the blisters are crusted over.

25. **What is an attack rate?**
An attack rate is somewhat akin to an incidence rate. Typically, attack rates are used for a specific group of people during a certain time period. It is often used to quantify epidemics.

$$\text{Primary attack rate} = \frac{\text{No. of people at risk in whom illness develops}}{\text{Total number of people at risk}}$$

An example of primary attack rate is the outbreak of *Salmonella* infection that occurred in October 2004 at a restaurant in East Oshkosh. Of the 200 patrons who ate there, 100 fell ill. Therefore the attack rate would be $100/200 = 50/100 = 0.5 = 50\%$

26. **One hundred school-aged children were exposed to varicella and 10 contracted chickenpox. The 10 children were forced to stay home with their younger, non-school-aged siblings, who had never been exposed to chickenpox. Unfortunately for the parents, of the 20 younger siblings, none of them had received the chickenpox vaccine; subsequently, 5 of them contracted chickenpox. Based on this information, what would the secondary attack rate be for this chickenpox outbreak?**
The secondary attack rate is a ratio: the number of new cases among contacts occurring within the accepted incubation period following exposure to a primary case divided by the total number of exposed contacts (i.e., person-to-person spread of the disease from primary cases to other persons). The formula for secondary attack rate is as follows:

$$\frac{\text{No. of cases who develop the disease within the incubation period}}{\text{No. of susceptible individuals who were exposed to the primary cases}}$$

The secondary attack rate of chickenpox among unvaccinated close contacts in this group of siblings would be 5/20, or 25%.

27. **What is an example of case-fatality ratio (CFR)?**
CFR is typically expressed as the percentage of individuals who are diagnosed with a certain disease and subsequently die because of that particular illness within a specified time period. For example, say that 1000 college students in Boston were infected with meningococcal meningitis. In 2003, 10 of the students died of complications directly related to the disease. Therefore, the case-fatality rate would be 10 deaths/1000 diagnosed cases, or a CFR of 1%, in 2003.

28. **How can I remember the difference between epidemic, endemic, and pandemic?**
You could try harkening back to your high school language classes and look at the base words:
- *Epi*demic: in Latin, *epi*-means "in addition." When defining an epidemic, one refers to the fact that each infected person is infecting multiple other individuals, so the number of infected persons is growing exponentially. In other words, each infected person is rapidly "adding" to the problem.
- *En*demic: the Latin meaning of this base is "in." Remember that endemic refers to a disease that is always present, to a greater or lesser extent, in folks who live "in/en" a particular geographic location.
- *Pan*demic: in Greek, *pan* means "all." A pandemic is an epidemic that is widespread over a large area or "all" of a geographic area. Recall that a *pan*oramic view is a view of the "big" picture or "all" of the geographic area.
  And, of course, remember that "-demic" is the root for "people" in Greek!

29. **So what is an epidemic in plain English?**
An epidemic is simply a higher frequency of disease or injury than is expected for a typical population and time period.

30. **What is an outbreak?**
Another term for epidemic.

KEY POINTS: DETECTION OF INFECTIOUS DISEASE

1. Always consider multisystem disease and review all confounders in diagnosing an infectious illness.

2. Put emergent treatable infectious diseases on the top of differential lists.

3. Physical, biologic, and occupational illnesses and chemical agents need to be considered in this potential bioterrorism-induced disease environment and era.

4. Unusual presentations of commonly known pathologic infectious diseases are common.

31. **Recalling that histograms are useful tools, you choose to plot the recent outbreak of influenza using this method. What would such a diagram be called in epidemiologic terms?**
The use of a histogram to illustrate the course of an epidemic (by plotting the number of cases by time of onset) is referred to as an epidemic curve. An epidemic caused by a

single common exposure (i.e., point-source epidemic) is often caused by contaminated food or water. The point-source epidemic curve has a sudden rise and fall, with a common incubation period for those affected (Fig. 5-5). Propagated epidemics, often spread by person-to-person contact, have a plateau, representing the overlap of exposures and incubation periods (Fig. 5-6). Uncontrolled propagated epidemics will have progressively taller peaks.

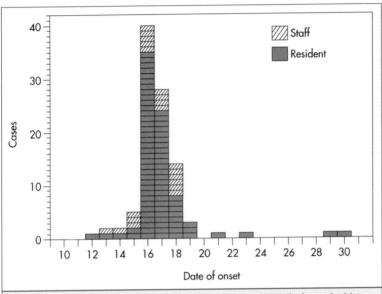

Figure 5-5. A point-source epidemic curve of an outbreak of influenza in a nursing home—Louisiana, August, 1993. (From CDC: Influenza A outbreaks—Louisiana, August, 1993. MMWR 42[36]:689–692, 1993.)

32. **What is the incubation period of a disease?**
It is the elapsed time of inapparent changes between exposure of the host to the infectious agent and the onset of the host's clinical illness. The incubation period is often a useful tool in determining the source of a point-source epidemic by back-calculating to determine the probable period of exposure of those affected to develop a list of likely causes.

33. **At 4:00 AM you are paged by the student health nurse at a local college, who states that 52 students in the waiting room are complaining of nausea, vomiting, and diarrhea of sudden onset. She fears an outbreak of *Salmonella* poisoning from the "chicken surprise" at the student dining hall last evening. What should you do?**
Initiate the 10 steps of an outbreak investigation listed below, as outlined by the Center for Disease Control and Prevention:
(1) Prepare for field work, (2) establish the existence of an outbreak, (3) verify the diagnosis, (4) define and identify cases, (5) describe and orient the data in terms of time, place, and person, (6) develop hypotheses, (7) evaluate hypotheses, (8) refine hypotheses and carry out additional studies, (9) implement control and prevention measures, and (10) communicate findings.

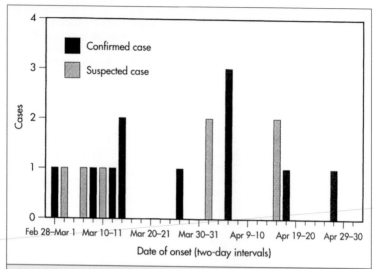

Figure 5-6. A propagated epidemic of *Escherichia coli (E. coli)* 0104:H21 infection resulting from continued exposure to contaminated milk—Helena, Montana, 1994. (From CDC: Outbreak of acute gastroenteritis attributable to *Escherichia coli* Serotype 0104:H21—Helena, Montana, 1994. MMWR 44[27]:501–504,

34. **A 62-year-old registered nurse in an acute care facility called the employee department, claiming she was diagnosed by her primary care physician with methicillin-resistant *Staphylococcus aureus* (MRSA) pneumonia. She was certain that she had acquired it from a patient who was just diagnosed as MRSA-positive. How can you tell if she contracted MRSA from that particular patient?**
Isolates of MRSA may be recovered from both the registered nurse and the patient. Genotyping, using pulsed-field gel electrophoresis (PFGE) testing, may then be performed on isolates from both individuals. If the PFGE patterns match, she has made her case.

35. **A health care worker presents in your office after a blood borne pathogen exposure to a source patient who is known to be hepatitis C-positive. You evaluate the worker, initiate treatment, and follow up as recommended by the CDC. You are interested in keeping a vigilant eye on this patient because of the source patient's history. What can you do, in addition to CDC recommendations, in terms of surveillance?**
An enhanced medical surveillance program may be useful in this setting for the following reasons:
- Up to 20% of hepatitis C conversions revert to no viral load.
- Early diagnosis is critical if reversion occurs; early counseling is critical if postexposure conversion happens because treatment within 6 months to a year improves outcome and prevents sustained viral response in 98% of health care workers.
- The enzyme-linked immunosorbent assay (ELISA) hepatitis C antibody test has a low specificity with a false-positive rate of up to 40%.
  Based on these facts, you may wish to obtain an antibody hepatitis C test at baseline and then order a polymerase chain reaction (PCR) viral RNA hepatitis C test and an antibody-hepatitis C test at 1, 3, and 6 months.

INFECTIOUS DISEASE USE IN BIOLOGIC WARFARE AND TERRORISM

36. **What characteristics of infectious diseases make them attractive for use in biologic warfare and terrorism?**
    Any or all of the below characteristics may make a particular infectious disease attractive:
    - Contagiousness
    - Incubation period
    - Viable methods of distribution (e.g., aerosolization)
    - Inadequate or complete lack of herd immunity
    - Mobile society, allowing rapid spread of disease beyond original area of distribution

37. **Which disease(s) listed below might be used in a bioterrorist attack?**
    - Smallpox
    - Anthrax
    - Bubonic plague
    - Q fever
    - Botulism
    - Tularemia
    - Viral hemorrhagic fever
    - Brucellosis

    According to the CDC, all of the agents listed have potential for use in biologic warfare.

38. **What organisms are considered by the CDC to be of the greatest threat with respect to bioterrorism?**
    The CDC designates organisms of this sort as category A. These agents include anthrax, plague, smallpox, tularemia, and viral hemorrhagic fevers, as well as botulinum toxin.

39. **What is syndromic surveillance?**
    According to the CDC Division of Public Health Surveillance and Informatics, syndromic surveillance is the process of collecting and interpreting health data that precede an actual diagnosis and may signal a case or outbreak that would trigger additional public health response.

40. **Why might schools be a good first source for epidemiologic evidence of a bioterrorist attack?**
    Using the premise of syndromic surveillance, a specified population, such as school children, may be monitored for symptoms related to exposure to infectious agents. Five-day-a-week required attendance, absence notification and recording, and, in many instances, the availability of school nurses to perform data collection make school children an excellent population for epidemiologic surveillance. In addition, school children may serve as efficient vectors for transmission of bioterrorism pathogens, with one child potentially infecting an entire family. Early detection of disease trends may lead to preemptive intervention strategies to avert a major disaster.

41. **How can I get real-time information about preparation and response to the use of infectious agents in terrorist events?**
    The CDC clinician registry for terrorism and emergency response provides updates on bioterrorism preparedness and training opportunities free to registered users at http://www.bt.cdc.gov/clinregistry/index.asp.

42. **Why are intermediate particles smaller than 5 μm important in aerosolization of infectious agents?**
    Particles smaller than 5 μm but greater than 1 μm will have the highest probability of transmitting infection. These intermediate-size particles can be respired more easily and deposited in the deep gas exchange regions of the lungs. Although particles greater than 5 μm are capable of transmitting infection via the pharynx or nasal cavity, they usually remain suspended and are removed upon exhalation. Suggested methods of aerosolization have included the use of crop dusters and entrainment into ambient air space through ventilation systems at offices and schools.

43. Why might infectious agents be more damaging than chemical agents?

Infectious agents have the ability to replicate, and some are contagious. Once chemical weapons have been released and decontamination is achieved, they no longer continue to expose a larger population. However, as in the case of smallpox, infectious agent transmission can continue until the last case is contained. Containment can be difficult because of varying incubation periods and individual immunogenicity.

44. How long can the smallpox (i.e., variola) virus remain viable outside the human host?

The variola virus can remain in a viable state on inanimate objects such as clothing and pillows for months. During the French and Indian War, the British distributed blankets infected with smallpox, which killed off almost 50% of the Indian tribes.

45. Since vaccinia is a live vaccine, can my patients develop smallpox from it?

No. Although vaccinia and smallpox are both orthopoxviruses, they are different organisms. While vaccinia can cause serious reactions such as generalized vaccinia, which may look similar to smallpox, it does not cause the actual disease.

WEBSITES

1. http://www.aidworkers.net/technical/ health/epidemiology.html.
2. http://www.brown.edu/Courses/Bio_160/Projects1999/av/mainpage.html.
3. http://www.bt.cdc.gov/Agent/agentlist.asp.
4. http://www.fda.gov/fdac/features/795_antibio.html.
5. http://www.syndromic.org/syndromicconference/2002/Supplementpdf/Pavlin.pdf.
6. http://www.niaid.nih.gov/factsheets/antimicro.htm.
7. http://nobelprize.org/medicine/laureates/1928/press.html.
8. http://www.microbeworld.org/htm/cissues/resist/resist_1.htm.
9. Wikipedia: http://en.wikipedia.org/wiki/World_War_I.

BIBLIOGRAPHY

1. Daigle CC, Chalupa DC, Gibb FR, et al: Ultrafine particle deposition in humans during rest and exercise. Inhal Toxicol 15(6):539–552, 2003.
2. Fenner F, Henderson DA, Arita I, et al. Smallpox and its Eradication. Geneva, Switzerland, World Health Organization, 1988.
3. Gates RA. Infectious Disease Secrets, 2nd ed. Philadelphia, Hanley & Belfus, 2003.
4. Jaeckel E. Treatment of hepatitis C with interferon alfa-2b. N Engl J Med 345:1252–1257, 2001.
5. MacFarlane J. Community-acquired pneumonia. Br J Dis Chest 81, 116–127, 1987.

CHAPTER 6

ISSUES IN ASSOCIATION AND CAUSATION

Christopher Jankosky, MD, MPH

1. **Are association and causation the same thing?**

   No. An association is a statistical relationship between two or more events, characteristics, or other variables. An additional level of evidence is required to support causation. Causation implies that a change in one variable is responsible, directly or indirectly, for an observed change in another variable.

2. **Do epidemiologic studies prove causation?**

   No. Epidemiologic studies cannot prove that causation occurs. Such studies, however, may be useful in supporting a causal association.

3. **An association between an exposure and an outcome can be due to what four mechanisms?**

   - **Spuriousness (i.e., artifact):** the association results from error or bias in the study design, implementation, or analysis.
   - **Confounding:** the relationship between an exposure and the development of a disease is distorted by an additional variable. In order to be a confounder, that additional variable must be associated with both the exposure and the disease. If confounders are recognized, adjustments can sometimes be used to minimize their impact.
   - **Chance:** there is always the possibility that an observed association is due to chance alone. For example, a *P* value of .05 corresponds to a 5% chance that the association is due to chance alone. Even when small *P* values are obtained, there is the possibility that an association does not truly exist and the relationship is pure chance.
   - **Causation:** An association due to a causal mechanism is generally determined after the above three mechanisms are addressed and criteria such as Hill's postulates are used. A causal association refers to a factor directly or indirectly causing an observed outcome.

4. **What is a risk factor?**

   A condition, element, or activity that may adversely affect an individual's health. It is consistently associated with the increased probability of developing a disease. On the other hand, protective factors are those conditions that lower the chances of a person developing a disease.

5. **Is a risk factor the same thing as a cause?**

   No. A patient's risk factors are only associated with an increased probability of developing a condition or disease. They do not necessarily imply a cause-and-effect relationship.

6. **How do epidemiologists quantify risk?**

   Epidemiologists often look at risk in terms of the following:

   - **Absolute risk:** the magnitude of the disease risk in a group of people with a specific exposure.
   - **Relative risk:** the strength of the association between an exposure and a disease.
   - **Attributable risk:** the proportion of disease risk that can be attributed to an exposure.

KEY POINTS: TYPES OF ASSOCIATION

1. Causation

2. Spuriousness (i.e., artifact)

3. Confounding

4. Chance

7. **What are two common study designs used for determining whether there is an association between a specific characteristic and a disease?**
The two most common designs are case-control and cohort. Both evaluate individual character-istics and are thus extremely useful in determining whether an association exists. For each individual subject, there is information about both the characteristic and the disease outcome. Since individual data matching is possible, robust analysis may be used to evaluate for confounding, effect modification, and bias. Studies of individual characteristics are therefore the most commonly used epidemiologic method for evaluating associations.

8. **What is an ecologic study?**
An ecologic study evaluates group characteristics in a population. The data used in these studies do not match any single individual to both risk factor and outcome; these studies contain data only on groups, or an entire population, often from large, centralized databases.
An example of an ecologic study is the association between rising rates of obesity and rising rates of diabetes in the United States. Although such a study does not demonstrate that those individuals who are obese are actually developing diabetes, it generates a hypothesis that can be pursued with a case-control or cohort study of individual characteristics.

9. **What is the ecologic fallacy?**
Ecologic studies evaluate group characteristics in a population. Because individuals are not followed, it is not possible to attribute a causal relationship to an observed association. For example, countries with a high average dietary fat intake also tend to have high rates of breast cancer. However, it is mostly industrialized countries that have both higher fat intakes and higher breast cancer rates. All of the other differences between industrialized and develop-ing countries cannot be taken into account. Therefore, many other potential causative factors are excluded.
Additionally, variability among individuals cannot be addressed. In the preceding example, we do not know if the individuals who developed breast cancer were the same as those who ate high-fat diets. It may be that those who developed breast cancer ate predominantly low-fat diets. Ecologic studies are valuable in suggesting areas for further research, but by themselves cannot demonstrate a causal relationship.

10. **Why is A. B. Hill frequently referenced in causation literature?**
A number of guidelines have been proposed to allow for critical evaluation when deriving causal inferences from epidemiologic studies. They rely on the use of all available information to estab-lish whether an association is causal. The most widely cited are often referred to as Hill's criteria.
A. B. Hill posed these criteria in 1965 as a list of standards, having adapted them from the U.S. Surgeon General's 1964 report on smoking and health. They serve as a general guide, and not all criteria must be fulfilled to establish causation. Although some of the criteria have been criticized in the past 40 years, they remain a reasonable framework through which to determine causal associations.

KEY POINTS: TYPES OF CAUSATION

1. Direct or indirect

2. Necessary and/or sufficient

3. Immediate or remote

11. **What are Hill's criteria for causality?**
    - **Strength of the association:** the stronger the association (e.g., relative risk or odds ratio), the more likely the relationship is causal.
    - **Consistency:** the association is repeatedly observed in studies performed by different persons, in different settings, among different populations, and using different methods.
    - **Specificity:** a specific exposure can be isolated from others and associated with a specific disease. This is perhaps the most difficult criterion to fulfill, because in practice many exposures (e.g., cigarettes or radiation) are associated with multiple effects and specific diseases often have more than one cause.
    - **Temporality:** the factor believed to have caused the disease must have occurred prior to disease development.
    - **Biologic gradient:** a dose-response relationship is present, so that as the exposure increases, either the risk of disease onset or the severity of disease also increases.
    - **Plausibility:** the relationship is explainable within the existing knowledge of the day. A. B. Hill recognized this as a criterion that we cannot demand, as there will be novel associations that uncover deficiencies in current biological thinking.
    - **Coherence:** the association does not seriously conflict with the natural history and biology of the disease process.
    - **Experimental evidence:** experiments support the association.
    - **Analogy:** examples of similar associations have been previously described for other disease entities.

    Hill AB: The environment and disease: Association or causation? Proc R Soc Med 58:295–330, 1965.

12 **What is the hierarchy of experimental evidence?**
    Not all experimental evidence carries the same weight. The hierarchy for epidemiologic research designs has four main groupings. From strongest to weakest, they are
    1. Randomized clinical trials
    2. Cohort studies
    3. Case-control studies and cross-section studies
    4. Case reports and case series

13. **What is the difference between direct and indirect causation?**
    Direct causation describes a causal pathway in which a factor directly causes a disease without any intermediate steps. Indirect causation describes a relationship in which a factor causes a disease through one or more intermediate steps. Because of the complex nature of human biology and physiology, there are almost always intermediate steps in epidemiologically observed relationships.

14. **What are the four types of causal relations?**
    - **Necessary and sufficient:** a factor is both necessary (i.e., disease will occur only if the factor is present), and sufficient (i.e., exposure always leads to disease). This type of relationship is rarely encountered.

- **Necessary but not sufficient:** more than one factor is required, usually in a temporal sequence. The initiation and promotion stages associated with carcinogenesis models is an example of this type of causal relation.
- **Sufficient but not necessary:** a specific factor can cause a disease process, but other factors by themselves can cause the same disease. For example, vitamin B_{12} deficiency can cause an anemia, but other factors can result in anemia as well.
- **Neither sufficient nor necessary:** a specific factor can be combined with other factors to produce a disease. However, the disease may be produced even in the absence of the factor. This is a causal model observed frequently in chronic diseases. For example, multiple risk factors for the development of atherosclerotic heart disease are neither sufficient nor necessary.

15. **What is confounding?**

Confounding occurs when the exposure-outcome association occurs solely because a distinct third factor is associated with both the exposure and the outcome. The observed association is true, but is not causal (see Fig. 6-1). A common example of confounding is the relationship among alcoholic beverage consumption, lung cancer, and cigarette smoking. Individuals who smoke more cigarettes tend to drink more alcoholic beverages, and individuals who smoke more cigarettes are at increased risk for lung cancer. Studies have revealed an association between alcoholic beverage consumption and lung cancer, although there is no causal link between them: cigarette smoking is a confounding factor. After controlling for cigarette smoking, the association between alcohol consumption and lung cancer disappears.

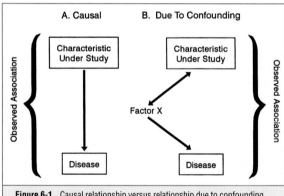

Figure 6-1. Causal relationship versus relationship due to confounding. (From Gordis L: Epidemiology, 3rd ed. St. Louis, Elsevier-Saunders, 2004.)

16. **List some methods to minimize confounding.**
- The study participants can be matched for the potential confounding variable (e.g., age or gender).
- Information can be collected on the potential confounding factor during the study, and its possible effect can be adjusted during analysis.
- The study can be restricted to a population group lacking the confounding factor, trait, or behavior.

17. **Explain effect modification.**

A factor that changes the strength of an association between two variables is known as an effect modifier. The interaction by the third factor, the effect modifier, will lead to a greater or lesser association than would be expected in its absence.

18. **What is synergism?**

Synergism is a type of effect modification. It refers to a situation in which two risk factors, when present together, result in an effect greater than a simple additive effect. For example, both cigarette smoking and asbestos exposure increase the risk of lung cancer. However, when an individual is exposed to both factors, the risk of lung cancer is far greater than would be expected by simply adding the two individual risks together. This concept is generally based on statistical considerations, and under ideal circumstances should be validated by biologic knowledge.

19. **Define bias.**

Bias is a systematic error in the design, implementation, or analysis of a study that results in an estimate that differs from the truth. Bias is not a simple error in calculation. For example, suppose a study design with an inherent bias was performed flawlessly by five different research institutions. The average of their results would still produce a mistaken estimate of an exposure's effect on the risk of disease.

20. **Give the two main categories of bias.**

Information bias and selection bias.

21. **What is information bias?**

Information bias results from flawed procedures in collecting data or imperfect definitions of study variables.

22. **What is selection bias?**

Selection bias can occur whenever an investigator selects his source population or determines eligibility criteria, or whenever conditions influence the subjects' choice to participate. Although, in some cases of selection bias, the internal validity of the study may be unaffected, it will affect the generalizability or external validity of the study.

Exclusion bias is a type of selection bias in which the investigators apply different eligibility criteria to the cases and the controls. For example, consider a study of drug abuse cases in an inner city emergency room. For a control population, the researches decide to use phone interviews of individuals whose addresses are within the same neighborhood. Such a study would exclude all of those who are homeless or do not have a phone.

Berkson's bias is another type of selection bias. It arises as a mathematic phenomenon when studies use hospital admission rates. Hospitalization rates for individuals with the target disease will differ from the rates of those with the control condition.

23. **What are four main types of information bias?**

- Misclassification bias
- Recall bias
- Reporting bias
- Surveillance bias

24. **Describe misclassification bias.**

Study participants may be mistakenly placed in the incorrect study group. For example, in a case-control study, some of the cases may be misclassified as controls and some of the controls may be misclassified as cases.

The bias may be introduced in a random fashion (i.e., nondifferential), as when one of several interviewers asks more probing questions of patients than the other interviewers do. In nondifferential misclassification, there is an error in the method of data collection that equally affects both the cases and the controls. This may balance out between the groups, diminishing the overall bias in the resulting association.

KEY POINTS: TYPES OF BIAS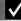

1. Information bias

2. Misclassification bias

3. Recall bias

4. Reporting bias

5. Surveillance bias

6. Selection bias

7. Exclusion bias

8. Lead-time bias

9. Berkson's bias

Or the bias could be systemic (i.e., differential), as when all the interviewers ask the case patients more probing questions than those asked of the controls. In differential misclassification, the rate of misclassification is higher in either the cases or controls, introducing the potential for significant error.

25. **Describe recall bias.**
Recall bias is a differential recall between cases and controls. A relevant piece of information may be recalled by the case patient, but forgotten by the control. There is a natural tendency for an individual with a disease to try to identify some unusual exposure which may have contributed to their condition, which often results in misclassification bias.

26. **Describe reporting bias.**
Reporting bias results when a larger percentage of either case or control subjects are reluctant to report an exposure due to attitudes, perceptions, or other concerns. Such withholding of information may also result in misclassification bias.

27. **Describe surveillance bias.**
Disease may be better ascertained in a monitored population than in the general population. The subpopulation of airplane pilots undergoes frequent and intensive routine medical evaluations. Some conditions may have a higher prevalence in pilots when compared to the overall population, in which routine surveillance is not performed.

28. **What is lead-time bias?**
It is recognized that medical screening will advance the date of diagnosis for a disease. Consider that, on average, women who are screened for breast cancer will have earlier stage disease than those who present outside of a screening program. Lead-time is defined as the difference in time between the date of diagnosis with screening and the date of diagnosis without screening.
Consider a new cancer therapy being tested on a screened group of patients. Unless lead time is accounted for, their survival time should not be compared to an unscreened control group of patients. Otherwise, the increase in survival time due solely to the advanced date of diagnosis will result in lead-time bias.

29. **What is the healthy worker effect?**
Subpopulations of workers will usually be healthier than those in the general population. Not only are the healthy more likely to obtain employment, but, once employed, they are more likely to have employer-based insurance, which improves access to health care compared to the unemployed. Thus, one must be careful when interpreting studies in which working populations are compared to general populations.

30. **When sample sizes are small, perhaps due to a rare exposure or disease, it may be difficult to have enough statistical power to demonstrate an association. Describe a method to address this issue.**
A quantitative systematic review, referred to as a meta-analysis, can be performed. The results of multiple studies that are considered combinable are aggregated to obtain a precise estimate of the relationship in question. Although meta-analysis cannot overcome the limitations and potential biases of the individual studies on which it is based, it can be a very useful method of clarifying an association.

WEBSITES

1. http://www.acepidemiology.org

2. http://www.apic.org

BIBLIOGRAPHY

1. Gordis L: Epidemiology, 2nd ed. Philadelphia, W.B. Saunders, 2000.

2. Greenberg RS, Daniels RD, Flanders WD, et al: Medical Epidemiology. New York, Lange Medical Books/McGraw-Hill, 2001.

3. Hill AB: The environment and disease: Association or causation? Proc R Soc Med 58:295–300, 1965.

4. Lilienfeld DE, Stolley PD: Foundations of Epidemiology, 3rd ed. New York, Oxford University Press, 1994.

5. Rothman KJ: Epidemiology: An Introduction. Oxford, Oxford University Press, 2002.

CHAPTER 7

RESEARCH MODEL DESIGNS

Ashita Tolwani, MD, MSc

1. **What is research design?**
   It is the specific approach best suited to answering a given research question.

2. **List the two basic design strategies used in epidemiologic research.**
   - Descriptive study design
   - Analytic study design

3. **What do descriptive studies describe?**
   The general characteristics of the distribution of a disease—or health condition—in relation to person, place, and time.

4. **What are analytic studies?**
   Analytic studies systematically evaluate suspected relationships between an exposure and a health outcome. Often they test hypotheses formulated from descriptive studies in order to determine whether a particular exposure causes or prevents disease. As a result, they usually provide stronger evidence concerning relationships.

5. **How are descriptive studies useful?**
   - They can help health care providers and administrators allocate resources efficiently.
   - They are useful in developing effective prevention and education programs.
   - They aid in formulating hypotheses that can be tested using an analytic design.

6. **Why are descriptive studies cheaper and faster than analytic studies?**
   They use information that is often routinely collected and easily available, such as data from production and sales, clinical records from hospitals, census data, and vital statistics records.

7. **List the types of descriptive studies.**
   - Correlation studies (e.g., studies of populations or ecologic studies)
   - Case reports
   - Case series
   - Cross-section surveys

8. **What are correlation studies?**
   Correlation studies use data from entire populations to compare disease frequencies either between different groups during the same period of time or in the same population at different points in time.

9. **What are the limitations of correlation studies?**
   Because correlation studies use data from whole populations rather than individuals, they cannot link an exposure to a disease occurrence in the same person. Another limitation is the inability to control for the effects of other factors that may be associated with the outcome. (These factors are also known as *confounders*.)

10. **Define a case report?**
A detailed description of the experience of a single patient.

11. **Define a case series?**
A case series describes the characteristics of a number of patients with a given disease, characteristic, or exposure.

12. **What are the limitations of case reports and case series?**
- Case reports are based on the experience of only one person; that is, the information is anecdotal.
- Case series lack an appropriate comparison group.

13. **What is a cross-section survey?**
A cross-section survey assesses the status of an individual with respect to the presence or absence of both exposure and disease at the same point in time. It provides a snapshot of the experience of a population at a specified time.

14. **List the strengths of a cross-section survey.**
- It provides estimates of prevalence of disease or other health outcomes.
- It can study entire populations or a representative sample.
- It provides greater ability to be generalized.

15. **List the limitations of a cross-sectional survey.**
- Since exposure and disease are assessed at the same time, the temporal relationship between an exposure and disease cannot be determined.
- It is subject to selection and observation bias (discussed below).

16. **List the two main types of analytic studies.**
- Observational studies
- Interventional studies (i.e., clinical trials)

17. **Describe the observational study format.**
Observational studies examine the association between risk factors and outcomes. The researchers do not interfere with or manipulate any of the factors of the study, but simply observe the natural course of events and explain what they observe with measures of association.

18. **Describe the interventional (i.e., experimental) study format.**
Interventional studies explore the association between interventions and outcomes. Researchers attempt to show that A causes B by manipulating specific factors that might have something to do with causing some outcome.

19. **What is the difference between the two types of studies (observational and interventional)?**
The active influence of exposure status by the researcher.

20. **What are the different types of observational studies?**
- Case-control studies
- Cohort studies

21. **What is a case-control study?**
In a case-control study, subjects who develop a condition (i.e., a disease) and subjects who have not developed a condition are selected, and the two groups are compared with respect to prior exposure. Subjects with the condition are called cases; subjects without the condition are controls.

22. Schematically represent the timing of initiation of the investigation for a case-control study in relation to exposure and outcome.
See Figure 7-1.

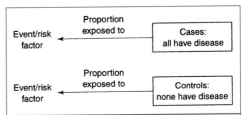

23. Give an example of a case-control study design.
To test the hypothesis that estrogen is a potential factor for uterine cancer, a group of women with uterine cancer (i.e., cases) and a group of women without uterine cancer who accurately reflect the population from which the cases have come (i.e., controls) are selected for evaluation. The use of estrogen by women in the case group is compared to the use of estrogen by women in the control group.

Figure 7-1. A typical case-control study. (From Vetter N, Matthews I: Epidemiology and Public Health Medicine. New York, Churchill Livingstone, 1999.)

24. What are the most important factors when choosing a control group in a case control study?
The risk factors of the control patients should be representative of those in the population "at risk" of becoming cases. In other words, control patients would have been included in the study as cases if they had the disease. Also, their exposures should be measurable with the same accuracy as those of cases.

25. List the strengths of case-control studies.
- Case-control studies are cheaper and faster, compared with other analytic designs.
- They are useful for studying diseases with long latent periods.
- They are useful for studying rare diseases since subjects are selected on the basis of disease status.
- They allow the investigation of multiple exposures simultaneously.

26. What are the limitations of case-control studies?
- They are not suited for evaluating rare exposure unless the study is very large or the exposure is common among those with the disease.
- Calculation of the incidence of disease in exposed and nonexposed groups cannot be performed unless the case-control study is population-based.
- The temporal relationship between exposure and disease cannot always be established.
- They are subject to bias (discussed below).

27. How does the analysis of case-control studies differ from other types of studies?
Because the rate of disease is unknown in case-control studies, the relative risk cannot be calculated. The odds ratio is used to estimate the relative risk.

28. When is the odds ratio a reasonable estimate for relative risk?
The odds ratio and relative risk are comparable in magnitude when the disease is rare.

29. What are cohort studies?
In a cohort study, subjects are defined by the presence or absence of an exposure to a suspected risk factor for a disease, and then they are followed over time.

30. What are some other names for cohort studies?
Longitudinal studies and prospective studies.

31. **Give the two types of cohort studies.**
    - Prospective
    - Retrospective

32. **What are the differences between prospective cohort studies and retrospective cohort studies?**
    - In a prospective cohort study, a group of subjects exposed to a risk factor (i.e., cases) is identified, along with a group of subjects not exposed (i.e., controls). The two groups are then followed prospectively and the incidence of disease in each group is measured.
    - In a retrospective cohort study, a group of subjects is identified in which the exposures and outcomes of interest have already occurred when the study is initiated; however, the exposures and outcomes are not a factor in subject grouping.

33. **Show schematics illustrating the difference between the design of prospective and retrospective cohort studies.**
    See Figures 7-2 and 7-3.

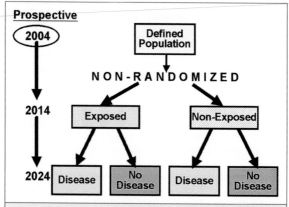

Figure 7-2. Time frame for a hypothetical prospective control study begun in 2004. (From Gordis L: Epidemiology, 3rd ed. Philadelphia, Elsevier-Saunders, 2004.)

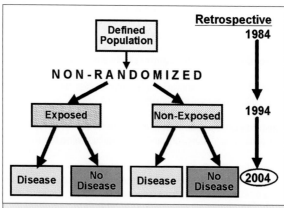

Figure 7-3. Time frame for a hypothetical retrospective cohort study begun in 2004. (From Gordis L: Epidemiology, 3rd ed. Philadelphia, Elsevier-Saunders, 2004.)

34. **Give an important factor in the design of a retrospective cohort study.**
    The choice of study subject must be made totally based on the exposure status, without knowledge of outcome.

35. **How should the exposed and unexposed groups be related in a cohort study?**
    The two groups should be similar in every way except for exposure status to the potential risk factor or factors.

36. **List the advantages of cohort studies.**
    - They are useful for studying rare exposures.
    - They can examine multiple effects of one exposure.
    - They can demonstrate a temporal association between exposure and disease.
    - They enable measurement of disease incidence in the exposed and nonexposed groups.

37. **List the limitations of cohort studies.**
    - Large, lengthy, and costly studies are required if the disease is rare or slow to develop.
    - If retrospective, they require the availability of records.
    - If cases are lost during the study, the loss may result in selection bias (discussed later).

38. **Describe the nested case-control study.**
    It is a type of case-control study that obtains its cases and controls from a cohort population that has been followed for a period of time.

39. **Provide a schematic of a nested case-control study.**
    See Figure 7-4.

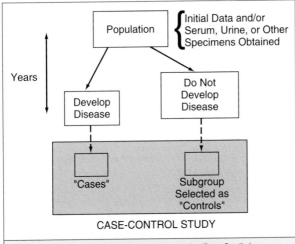

Figure 7-4. Diagram of a nested case-control study. (From Gordis L: Epidemiology, 3rd ed. Philadelphia, Elsevier-Saunders, 2004.)

40. **What are interventional trials?**
    A treatment or preventive intervention is provided to a group of subjects; their subsequent experiences are compared to those of subjects not given the intervention.

41. What is the basic strategy behind an experimental study?
To show that a treatment is effective, the improvement rate in a treated group should be greater than the improvement rate in an untreated group. In addition, it should be unlikely that the differences in rates are caused by chance alone.

42. How should the control group be related to the treatment group?
The control group should be similar to the treatment group in all characteristics associated with the expected outcome—except that they should not receive the studied treatment. The control group may be receiving the standard treatment for the risk factor or, instead, a placebo.

43. List the types of interventional trials.
- Randomized controlled trial (RCT)
- Quasi-experimental trial

44. What is an RCT?
It is a study design used to evaluate the effectiveness of interventions (e.g., pharmacologic treatments and diagnostic tests). An RCT consists of one treatment group and one control group. The treatment group receives the treatment under investigation while the control group receives either no treatment of some current standard treatment. Patients are randomly assigned to the groups.

45. Why do we need RCTs to evaluate treatments?
When RCTs are sufficiently large and carefully designed, they can provide the strongest evidence for the existence of a cause-effect relationship.

46. What is the purpose of randomization?
Random allocation helps ensure that the groups in clinical trials are comparable. Each subject has an equal chance of being assigned to either group in the study, so that both groups are similar in all characteristics (e.g., gender, age, race, and severity of disease) that may affect the outcome.

47. Does randomization guarantee the groups are comparable?
No. Chance may play a role in making the groups not comparable. The effect of this random error can be reduced by using a large enough sample size.

48. Represent a randomized trial design schematically.
See Figure 7-5.

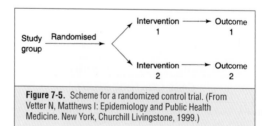

Figure 7-5. Scheme for a randomized control trial. (From Vetter N, Matthews I: Epidemiology and Public Health Medicine. New York, Churchill Livingstone, 1999.)

49. In the previous schematic, what are the four possible outcomes?
1. The treatments do not differ, and we correctly conclude that they do not differ.
2. The treatments do not differ, but we incorrectly conclude that they differ.

3. The treatments differ, but we incorrectly conclude that they do not differ.
4. The treatments differ, and we correctly conclude that they differ.

50. **What are the advantages of RCTs?**
    - Their design is prospective.
    - They eliminate bias by comparing two otherwise identical groups.

51. **What are the disadvantages of RCTs?**
    They are relatively expensive and time-consuming.

52. **What is bias?**
    Bias (i.e., systematic error) is an error in a study that results in an incorrect assessment of the association between exposure and risk of disease.

53. **List the two major types of bias.**
    - Selection bias
    - Observation (i.e., information) bias

54. **Is random error a form of bias?**
    No. Random error occurs by chance.

55. **What is selection bias?**
    Selection bias occurs when study participants are selected in such a way that the association between exposure and disease differs for those who participate and those who do not participate in the study.

56. **List the different ways selection bias can occur.**
    - Selection of an inappropriate comparison group by the investigator
    - Self-selection by the subject (i.e., volunteering)
    - Nonresponse by the subject (i.e., refusal)
    - Losing track of subjects during the study
    - Subjects die during the study

57. **Which types of studies are susceptible to selection bias?**
    - Case-control studies
    - Cross-section studies
    - Cohort studies (selection bias is least common in cohort studies)

58. **Give an example of selection bias.**
    Suppose that the efficacy of a new screening test to detect cancer was assessed in the community by comparing the incidence rate of cancer among those who volunteered to be tested with the incidence rate among community members who were not tested. Such a comparison suffers from selection bias since the subjects who volunteer for cancer screening may differ from those who do not volunteer. For example, those who volunteer may be more health conscious than those who do not volunteer: volunteers may have a diet and exercise regimen that reduces the risk of cancer and, thus, might be expected to have a lower rate of cancer.

59. **How does observation bias occur?**
    Observation bias is a systematic error that occurs because the information collected about the study subjects is erroneous. Inaccurate or incomplete data can lead to incorrect associations.

60. **List the types of observation bias?**
    - Recall bias
    - Interviewer bias
    - Misclassification bias

KEY POINTS: RESEARCH MODEL DESIGNS

1. The two basic epidemiologic design strategies are the descriptive study design and the analytic study design.

2. Descriptive studies examine the distribution of diseases in populations; analytic studies examine the determinants of diseases in populations.

3. Descriptive studies include correlation studies, case reports, case series, and cross-section surveys.

4. Analytic studies include observational studies and interventional studies.

5. Observational studies examine how exposure to risk factors influences the probability of developing disease; in interventional studies, the investigator controls which treatment each subject receives.

6. Observational studies include cohort and case-control studies and are subject to selection and observation bias.

7. Randomized controlled trials, a type of interventional study, provide the most reliable evidence of treatment effectiveness.

61. **Define each type of observation bias.**
    - **Recall bias** occurs when subjects with a particular condition or disease remember their previous exposure experience differently from those who do not have the disease.
    - **Interviewer bias** occurs when the investigator obtains or interprets the information differently from those with the health condition and those without the health condition.
    - **Misclassification bias** occurs when errors are made in the categorization of either exposure or disease status.

62. **Give an example of recall bias.**
    Suppose a study is done to obtain exposure information on birth malformations by interviewing women who have had babies with birth malformations and women who have not had babies with birth malformations. Mothers who have given birth to babies with birth malformations are more likely to remember details about exposures, such as medications taken, because they are highly motivated to find out why their babies were born with malformations. Mothers who have experienced normal births have no compelling reason to remember such details and may forget these exposures.

63. **What is the study design for the above question?**
    Case-control.

64. **Why is bias more problematic in case-control studies than in any other analytic design?**
    Since both the exposure and the outcome have already occurred when information is obtained on the study patients, knowledge of the exposure status can influence the selection of individuals into the study, resulting in selection bias. Also, the knowledge of the disease status can

influence the way information on the exposure is reported by the subjects or the investigator, causing recall bias and interviewer bias.

65. **What is blinding in a study?**
Blinding occurs when the treatment assignment is hidden from the subject but not the observer.

66. **What is meant by double-blinding and triple-blinding?**
Double-blinding means neither the observer nor the subject is aware of the treatment assignment. Triple-blinding means the observer, the subject, and the individual administering the treatment are not aware of the treatment assignments.

67. **What is the purpose of blinding?**
The purpose of blinding is to minimize the possibility of observation bias in determining the outcome.

68. **What is confounding?**
A confounder is a factor that is associated both with the exposure of interest and with the risk of developing the disease. Thus, the observed association between the exposure of interest and disease outcome may be incorrect. Confounding also causes error in comparisons between groups if the groups are not truly comparable due to differences in age, gender, health status, and other risk factors.

69. **Give an example of confounding.**
Suppose an investigator is studying the relationship between a certain medication and death. The study demonstrates a relationship between the use of the medication and an increased risk of death. However, age is an additional factor that can affect the observed association. Older people have an increased risk of death compared to younger people. In this example, age confounds the relationship between the use of the medication and risk of death.

70. **What methods can be used in the study design to control for confounding?**
- Randomization
- Restriction
- Matching

71. **Describe how the three methods listed above control for confounding.**
- **Randomization** has already been discussed above and is applicable only to interventional studies. With a large enough sample size, randomization allows for all potential confounders, including those unknown to the investigator, to be evenly distributed between the treatment groups.
- **Restriction** involves limiting the selection of subjects to those who have the same value as the factor that may be a confounder. For example, if gender is a potential confounder, the selection of study subjects can be limited to a specific gender.
- **Matching** involves selecting patients so that the potential confounders are identically distributed between the treatment groups. For example, if age and gender are confounders, then for each patient of a certain age and gender in the diseased group, a patient of the same age and gender is selected in the control group.

72. **What are the disadvantages of matching?**
- It can be difficult, time-consuming, and expensive to find a comparison subject with all the appropriate matching characteristics for each subject in the study.
- The effect of the matched characteristic on outcome cannot be determined.
- Matching does not control for the effect of potential confounding factors for which matching was not done.

73. **What is a meta-analysis?**

It is a systematic review using statistical methods to combine and summarize the results of several studies.

74. **What is the hierarchy of study designs based on evidence?**
- **Level I: RCTs** are generally accepted as the most reliable evidence of whether a treatment is effective.
- **Level II: case-control or cohort trials**
  1. The next-best studies are well-designed case-control or cohort trials that are prospective, compare similar groups, and correct for confounding in the analysis.
  2. Less preferable are poorly designed case-control or cohort trials—ones that are retrospective, compare poorly matched groups, or make no attempt to correct for confounding.
- **Level III: case series** or other studies with no control groups.

BIBLIOGRAPHY

1. Altman DG: Practical Statistics for Medical Research. London: Chapman & Hall, CRC, 1990.
2. Gordis L: Epidemiology, 3rd ed. Philadelphia, Elsevier-Saunders, 2004.
3. Greenberg RS, Daniels SR, Flanders WD, et al: Medical Epidemiology, 3rd ed. New York, Lange Medical Books / McGraw Hill, 2001.
4. Hennekens CH, Buring JE: Epidemiology in Medicine. Philadelphia, Lippincott Williams & Wilkins, 1987.
5. Jekel JF, Katz DL, Elmore JG: Epidemiology, Biostatistics, and Preventive Medicine, 2nd ed. Philadelphia, W.B. Saunders, 2001.
6. Rothman KJ: Epidemiology: An Introduction. Oxford, Oxford University Press, 2002.
7. Vetter N, Matthews I: Epidemiology and Public Health Medicine. New York, Churchill Livingstone, 1999.

CHAPTER 8

EVIDENCE–BASED MEDICINE

Lee Okurowski, MD, MPH, MBA

1. **What is evidence-based medicine (EBM)?**
   EBM is an approach to medicine that integrates the current best evidence, clinical expertise, and patient values to optimize clinical outcomes and quality of life. With EBM comes the recognition that intuition, unsystematic clinical experience, and speculative pathophysiologic rationale are insufficient grounds for clinical decision-making. Instead, EBM maintains that a hierarchy of best research evidence exists. It is this best research evidence, based on clinically relevant research, that is to serve as the foundation for clinical decision making.

2. **When and how did EBM first develop?**
   The roots of EBM date to the late 1970s, when a group of clinical epidemiologists, led by David Sackett and his colleagues at McMaster University, began preparing a series of articles advising clinicians how to read clinical journals and apply evidence from the literature to direct patient care.

3. **Who first used the term *evidence-based medicine*?**
   The term was first used by Gordon Guyatt, MD, in 1990 while serving as residency director of the internal medicine program at McMaster.

4. **How are research, clinical expertise, and patient values related in EBM?**
   EBM recognizes that research evidence is never the sole determinant of clinical decision-making. Research evidence must be combined with clinical expertise to identify each individual patient's health state and diagnosis. An understanding of patient values is also necessary so that the unique preferences, concerns, and expectations that each patient brings to a clinical encounter can be integrated so that optimum clinical decision making can be achieved.

5. **What constitutes the evidence in EBM?**
   In EBM, any empirical observation about the relationship between event and clinical outcome constitutes potential evidence. Nonetheless, all evidence should not be viewed as equal in making clinical decisions.

6. **What is the hierarchy of evidence used in EBM?**
   The strength of evidence provided by the unsystematic observations of an individual clinician should not be viewed the same as the evidence provided by systematic and controlled clinical trials. An example of a hierarchy of strength of evidence for treatment decisions is listed, from most preferable to least, as follows:
   1. N of 1 randomized controlled trials
   2. A systematic review of randomized controlled trials
   3. A single randomized trial
   4. A systematic review of observation studies
   5. A single observational study
   6. Physiologic studies
   7. An unsystematic clinical observation

Guyatt GH, Haynes B, Jaeschke R, et al: Introduction: The philosophy of evidence-based medicine. In Guyatt GH, Rennie D (eds): Users' Guides to the Medical Literature: A Manual for Evidence-Based Clinical Practice. Chicago, American Medical Association, 2002, pp 5–20.

7. **How does the hierarchy of evidence rank randomized controlled studies versus observational studies? How does it rank multiple studies versus single studies?**

   The hierarchy demonstrates that, in general, the strength of evidence increases with randomized controlled studies, compared with observational studies. The hierarchy also demonstrates that the strength of evidence increases with multiple studies, compared to individual studies.

8. **What must clinicians remember when generalizing results from studies to individual patients?**

   When considering available research evidence in making decisions about the treatment of their patients, clinicians most often generalize results from studies of other people, which can weaken causal inferences about treatment effectiveness; clinicians must remember that there are still important questions to be answered about the applicability of research findings from the study group to the treatment of an individual patient outside the study.

9. **How is the N of 1 randomized controlled trial conducted?**

   An individual patient undergoes pairs of treatment periods: the patient receives an experimental treatment in one period of each of the paired treatment periods and a placebo or alternative treatment in the other period. If feasible, the clinician and patient are blinded to the allocation of treatment and the order of treatment is randomized. Typically, clinicians and patients make quantitative ratings of outcomes, and treatment periods are then alternated until the clinician and the patient are convinced that the patient is, or is not, receiving benefit from the experimental treatment.

10. **What are the strengths and weaknesses of N of 1 randomized controlled clinical trials?**

    The strengths are that they provide definitive evidence of effectiveness in individual patients, they are feasible, and they can lead to long-term changes in treatment administration and effects.

    Weaknesses include the fact that such trials require a high degree of interest, time, and cooperation between clinician and patient. N of 1 trials are not usually appropriate for short-term problems, therapeutic cures, determining long-term outcomes, or disorders that are rare.

Guyatt GH, Keller JL, Jaeschke R, et al. The n-of-1 randomized control trial: Clinical usefulness. Our three-year experience. Ann Intern Med 112:293–299, 1990.

Mahon J, Laupacis A, Donner A, Wood T: Randomised study of n of 1 trials versus standard practice. BMJ 312:1069–1074, 1996.

11. **What is the difference between background and foreground questions in EBM?**

    One of most difficult aspects of applying EBM to clinical practice is formulating answerable clinical questions for which there are best current evidence available. EBM considers clinical questions in two broad categories: background and foreground questions. Background questions ask for general knowledge about a disorder and attempt to answer the who, what, when, where, why, and how of the disorder or an aspect of the disorder. Foreground questions ask for specific information about managing patients with a disorder and typically ask about the patient, the problem, interventions, and clinical outcomes. Generally, as experience with a disorder increases, the clinician moves from asking a preponderance of background questions to foreground questions.

12. **What are the best sources for finding current best evidence?**
Electronic evidence databases, evidence-based journals, and online services are sources that provide significant current best evidence. These sources sharply contrast traditional medical textbooks, which are often not the most appropriate method of finding current best evidence. Although most medical textbooks often provide useful information on pathophysiology, they typically become quickly out-of-date with regard to information on cause, diagnosis, prognosis, prevention, and treatment of a given disorder.

13. **List some online resources that are particularly useful for evidence-based medicine.**
See Table 8-1.

TABLE 8-1.	ONLINE RESOURCES PARTICULARLY USEFUL FOR EVIDENCE-BASED MEDICINE
Resource	**URL**
ACP Journal Club	http://www.acpjc.org
ACP Medicine	http://www.acpmedicine.com
Best Bets	http://www.bestbets.org/
Centre for Evidence-Based Medicine	http://www.cebm.net/index.asp
Clinical Evidence	http://www.clinicalevidence.org/
Clinical practice guidelines	http://www.guidelines.gov
Cochrane Library	http://www3.interscience.wiley.com/ cgi-bin/mrwhome/106568753/HOME
emedicine	http://www.emedicine.com
Evidence-Based Medicine Reviews (OVID)	http://www.ovid.com
Evidence-Based	http://cebm.jr2.ox.ac.uk
Harrisons Online	http://www.harrisonsonline.com
London Links journal listings	http://www.londonlinks.ac.uk
MD Consult	http://www.mdconsult.com
Medical Matrix	http://www.medmatrix.org
Medline/PubMed	http://www.pubmed.gov
Medscape	http://www.medscape.com
ScHarr Netting the Evidence	http://www.shef.ac.uk/~scharr/ir/netting
United Health Foundation	http://www.unitedhealthfoundation.org
UpToDate	http://www.uptodate.com
WebMD	http://www.webmd.com

14. **What are the steps in conducting a general search strategy?**
1. Determine the clinical problem.
2. Define an important searchable and answerable question for the clinical problem of interest.
3. Determine the most likely evidenced resources.
4. Design a search strategy.
5. Summarize the evidence.
6. Apply the evidence.

15. **When using an article on the medical literature to answer clinical question, what are three questions that should always be asked?**
    1. Are the results of the study valid?
    2. Is the evidence important?
    3. How can the valid and important results be applied to patient care?

16. **What are the principal areas of patient care to which the tools of EBM are most frequently applied?**
    1. Diagnosis and screening
    2. Prognosis
    3. Therapy
    4. Harm

17. **You are reviewing the results of an article on a new screening test for thyroid cancer. The study was performed on a total of 2500 patients, of which 800 were eventually determined by surgical biopsy to have thyroid cancer and 1700 were determined by surgical biopsy to be disease-free. The new screening test was positive in 1000 patients, but only 750 of those who tested positive were eventually found to be positive on surgical biopsy. Construct a 2 × 2 table and determine the following: sensitivity, specificity, likelihood ratio positive (LR +), likelihood ratio negative (LR−), positive predictive value, negative predictive value, prevalence, pretest odds, posttest odds, and posttest probability.**

	Disease +	Disease −	Totals
Test+	750 [A]	250 [B]	1000 [A + B]
Test−	50 [C]	1450 [D]	1500 [C + D]
Totals	800 [A + C]	1700 [B + D]	2500 [A + B + C + D]

- Sensitivity = A/(A + C) = 750/800 = 94%
- Specificity = D/(B + D) = 1450/1700 = 85%
- LR+ = sensitivity/(1 − specificity) = 94%/15% = 6.27
- LR− = (1 − sensitivity)/specificity = 6%/85% = 0.07
- Positive predictive value = A/(A + B) =750/1000 = 75%
- Negative predictive value = D/(C + D) =1450/1500 = 97%
- Prevalence = (A + C)/(A + B + C + D) = 800/2500 = 32%
- Pretest odds = prevalence/(1 − prevalence) =32%/68% = 47%
- Posttest odds = pretest odds × likelihood ratio = 0.47 × 6.27 = 2.9
- Posttest probability = posttest odds/(posttest odds + 1) = 2.9/3.9 = 74%

18. **A patient presents for evaluation of a thyroid disorder and you suspect that she may have about a 50:50 chance of having thyroid cancer prior to applying the screening test. You apply the screening test and she tests positive. What are the patient's pretest odds?**
    A 50:50 chance translates to pretest odds of 1:1; therefore, the patient's pretest odds are 1.

19. **What are the patient's posttest odds?**
    To determine the posttest odds, the pretest odds of 1 are multiplied by the LR+ of 6.27; 1 × 6.27 = 6.27).

20. **What is the posttest probability?**
    The posttest probability = posttest odds/(posttest odds + 1). So the posttest probability = 6.27/(6.27 + 1) = 6.27/7.27 = 86.2%.

21. **What is the likelihood ratio positive (LR+)?**
The LR+ is simply the quotient of the sensitivity over the false positive rate. Note that both of these terms are not influenced by the prevalence; therefore, neither is the LR+.

22. **Why does a high LR+ make a given test more predictive?**
A high sensitivity is a desired quality of a test that is used to rule out those with negative results; sensitivity constitutes the numerator of the LR+ quotient. The false positive rate, 1 − specificity, serves as the denominator. Clearly, false positives are not desired because they wrongly "rule in" those without the disease state of interest. Putting it all together, maximizing the desired characteristic and minimizing the undesired will increase the LR+ quotient and, thus, the posttest probability.

23. **What is the likelihood negative ratio (LR−)?**
The quotient of the false-negative rate divided by the specificity. Using the same logic as above, one can qualitatively appreciate that a low LR− is desired because this ratio represents "missed cases" (i.e., false negatives) over appropriately "ruled in" cases.

24. **Can the LR+ and LR− give an indication of how useful a test is?**
Yes. We have determined that a useful test should have a high LR+ and a low LR−. One can therefore get an idea of the strength of a test by looking at the ratio of LR+/LR−. The higher the number, the better the test. In the example problem, the LR+/LR− is 6.27/0.07 which equals 89.6. There is no firm rule, but typically a LR+/LR− ratio greater than 50 is considered acceptable.

25. **Why are tests with very high values of sensitivity and specificity useful?**
Diagnostic tests with very high sensitivity values are useful for ruling out a given disease or condition when the results are negative. This can be remembered by the mnemonic **SnNout**: a **Sn**ensitive test with a **N**egative result rules **out** a disease. Diagnostic tests with a very high specificity values are useful for ruling in a given disease or condition when the results are positive. This can be remembered by the mnemonic **SpPin**: a **Sp**ecific test with a **P**ositive result rules **in** a disease.

26. **Describe the accuracy limitations of using sensitivity and specificity of diagnostic tests in determining patients with or without a given disorder. What statistical measures can be used to overcome these limitations?**
Sensitivity and specificity of a test are typically constrained to test results that are dichotomous (i.e., either positive or negative). As a result, the accuracy of many tests that have values along a continuum of values can be lost. The limitations of the traditional sensitivity and specificity can be overcome by comparing likelihood ratios across different levels of test results.

27. **Table 8-2 presents results of ventilation-perfusion (V/Q) scanning to determine the presence of pulmonary embolism. Calculate the likelihood ratios across each of the different levels of scan test results in patients with a pulmonary embolism versus a patient without a pulmonary embolism. Interpret these results.**
See Table 8-3.

28. **How do these likelihood ratios help clinically?**
The likelihood ratios provide a measure of how much a diagnostic test will raise or lower the pretest probability in determining the posttest probability for a given disease or disorder. A likelihood ratio of 1 means that the pretest probability and posttest probability are equal. Likelihood ratios greater than 1.0 increase the pretest probability that disease is present; the higher the likelihood ratio, the greater the increase in probability from the pretest probability to

TABLE 8-2. VENTILATION PERFUSION (V/Q) SCAN RESULTS

Pulmonary Embolism	Present	Absent	Likelihood Ratio
Scan Results	#	#	
High Probability	100	15	?
Intermediate Probability	105	215	?
Low Probability	40	270	?
Normal	5	125	?
Total	250	625	

TABLE 8-3. VENTILATION PERFUSION (V/Q) SCAN RESULTS

Pulmonary Embolism	Present	Proportion	Absent	Proportion	Likelihood Ratio
Scan Results	#		#		
High Probability	100	100/250=0.40	15	15/625=0.02	20
Intermediate Probability	105	105/250=0.42	215	215/625=0.34	1.2
Low Probability	40	40/250=0.16	270	270/625=0.43	0.37
Normal	5	5/250=0.02	125	125/625=0.20	0.10
Total	250		625		

the posttest probability. Likelihood ratios less than 1.0 decrease the pretest probability that disease is present; the lower the likelihood ratio, the lesser the increase in probability from the pretest probability to the posttest probability.

Data adapted from the Prospective Investigation of Pulmonary Embolism Diagnosis (PIOPED) investigators. Value of ventilation/perfusion scan in acute pulmonary embolism. Results of PIOPED. JAMA 263:2753–2759, 1990.

29. **What is a likelihood nomogram?**
   A likelihood nomogram, as displayed in Figure 8-1, is a graphical method for converting pretest to posttest probability using likelihood ratios.

30. **How is a likelihood nomogram used?**
   The left-hand column of numbers (*see* Fig. 8-1) displays the range of pretest probabilities, the middle column displays the likelihood ratios, and the right-hand column displays the posttest probabilities. To use the likelihood nomogram, start with the pretest probability and draw a straight line through the corresponding likelihood ratio to obtain the posttest probability.

31. **If a patient has a pretest probability of 50% for a pulmonary embolism, and also has a ventilation-perfusion scan of high probability, what is the patient's posttest probability, using the likelihood nomogram?**
   Drawing a straight line from a pretest probability of 50% through a likelihood ratio of 20.0 demonstrates a posttest probability of approximately 95%.

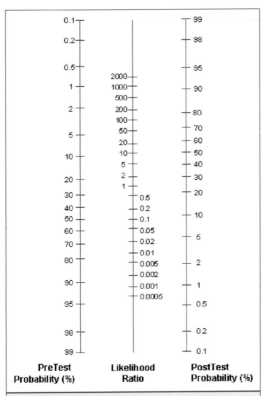

Figure 8-1. Likelihood nomogram. (From the Centre for Evidence-Based Medicine:http://www. cebm.net/likelihood_ratios. asp#example.)

32. What is meant by the term number needed to treat (NNT)?
The NNT is a numerical expression of the number of patients needed to receive an active treatment to demonstrate a benefit over no treatment and prevent one bad outcome. It is a helpful measure used in making medical decisions about an individual patient when summarizing results of clinical trials.

33. How is the NNT calculated?
The NNT is the inverse of the absolute risk reduction (ARR) and is given by the expression

$$NNT = 1/ARR$$
$$ARR = ARC - ART$$

where ARC = attributable risk control and ART = attributable risk treatment group, Expressed in these terms, NNT then becomes

$$NNT = 1 / (ARC - ART)$$

Chatellier G, Zapletal E, Lemaitre D, et al: The number needed to treat: A clinically useful nomogram in its proper context. BMJ 321:426–429, 1996.

KEY POINTS: EVIDENCE-BASED MEDICINE (EBM)

1. EBM integrates the current best evidence, clinical expertise, and patient values to optimize clinical outcomes and quality of life.

2. EBM recognizes that the strength of evidence provided by the unsystematic observations of an individual clinician should not be viewed the same as the evidence provided by systematic and controlled clinical trials. In general, the strength of evidence increases with randomized controlled studies compared with that of observation studies.

3. Electronic evidence databases, evidence-based journals, and online services are sources that most often provide the current best evidence.

4. When using an article in the medical literature to answer clinical questions, three useful questions should always be asked: (1) Are the results of the study valid? (2) Is the evidence important? and (3) How can the valid and important results be applied to patient care?

5. The tools of EBM are most frequently applied in examining clinical issues related to diagnosis and screening, prognosis, therapy, and harm.

34. **What are the key questions that must be considered when evaluating studies of diagnosis and screening?**
    1. Are the results of the study valid?
       - Was there diagnostic uncertainty across the spectrum of disease states?
       - Was the comparison blinded and was a gold standard for diagnosis applied across both treatment and control groups?
       - Was the gold standard applied regardless of the results of the diagnostic test being evaluated?
    2. Is the valid evidence important?
       - Was the valid evidence obtained by the diagnosis or screening test able to accurately distinguish patients with and without disease?
    3. How can the valid and important results be applied to patient care?
       - Is the diagnostic or screening test available, affordable, acceptable, accurate, and precise?
       - Is it possible to make sensible estimates of pretest probabilities for individual patients?
       - Will the subsequent posttest probabilities affect management or treatment?

Jaeschke R, Guyatt GH, Lijmer J: Diagnostic tests. In Guyatt GH, Rennie D (eds): Users' Guides to the Medical Literature: A Manual for Evidence-Based Clinical Practice. Chicago, American Medical Association, 2002, pp 187–217.

Sackett DL, Straus S, Richardson S, et al: Evidence-based Medicine: How to Practice and Teach EBM, 2nd ed. London, Churchill Livingstone, 2000, pp 67–94.

35. **What are the key questions that must be considered when evaluating studies of prognosis?**
    1. Are the results of the study valid?
       - Was a representative sample of patients assembled?
       - Are the patients homogeneous with respect to prognostic risk?
       - Was follow-up sufficiently long and complete?
       - Were objective, unbiased outcome criteria applied in a blind fashion?
    2. Is the valid evidence important?
       - How likely are the observed outcomes over time?
       - How precise are the estimates of prognosis?

3. How can the valid and important results be applied to patient care?
   - Are individual patients similar to those under study?
   - Will the evidence make a clinically relevant impact on patient care?

Randolph A, Bucher H, Richardson WS, et al: Prognosis. In Guyatt GH, Rennie D (eds): Users' Guides to the Medical Literature: A Manual for Evidence-Based Clinical Practice. Chicago, American Medical Association, 2002, pp 219–240.

Sackett DL, Straus S, Richardson S, et al: Evidence-based Medicine: How to Practice and Teach EBM, 2nd ed. London, Churchill Livingstone, 2000, pp 95–104.

36. **What are the key questions that must be considered when evaluating studies of therapy?**
    1. Are the results of the study valid?
       - Were patients randomized?
       - Were patients and clinicians blinded?
       - Was follow-up sufficiently long and complete?
       - Were patients analyzed throughout the study in their respective initial randomization groups?
       - Were groups treated equally except for the therapy under study?
    2. Is the valid evidence important?
       - What is the magnitude of the treatment effect?
       - How precise are the estimates of the treatment effect?
    3. How can the valid and important results be applied to patient care?
       - Are individual patients similar to those under study?
       - Will the therapy make a clinically relevant impact on patient care?
       - What are the potential benefits, harms, and costs of therapy?

Guyatt GH, Cook D, Devereaux PJ, et al: Therapy. In Guyatt GH, Rennie D (eds): Users' Guides to the Medical Literature: A Manual for Evidence-Based Clinical Practice. Chicago, American Medical Association, 2002, pp 81–120.

Sackett DL, Straus S, Richardson S, et al: Evidence-based Medicine: How to Practice and Teach EBM, 2nd ed. London, Churchill Livingstone, 2000, pp 105–154.

37. **What are the key questions that must be considered in evaluating studies of harm?**
    1. Are the results of the study valid?
       - Were patient groups clearly defined and was similarity defined in all important aspects of outcome?
       - Were any differences between groups adjusted for in the analysis?
       - Was follow-up sufficiently long and complete for the outcome to occur?
       - Were outcomes and exposures measured similarly among comparison groups?
       - Did the study meet necessary criteria for the establishment of causation?
    2. Is the valid evidence important?
       - What is the magnitude of the association of exposure and outcome?
       - What is the precision of the association of the exposure and outcome?
    3. How can the valid and important results be applied to patient care?
       - Are individual patients similar to those under study?
       - What are the benefits of treatment?
       - Are there alternatives to treatment?
       - What are the patient's risks for an adverse event?
       - Have the patient's preferences, concerns, and expectations been adequately considered?

WEBSITE (See also Table 8.1)

http://www.aso.org

BIBLIOGRAPHY

1. Dalla Vecchia LK, Grosfeld JL, West KW, et al: Intestinal atresia and stenosis: A 25-year experience with 277 cases. Arch Surg 133:490–496, 1998.

2. Guyatt GH, Haynes B, Jaeschke R, et al: Introduction: The philosophy of evidence-based medicine. In Guyatt GH, Rennie D (eds): Users' Guides to the Medical Literature: A Manual for Evidence-Based Clinical Practice. Chicago, American Medical Association, 2002, pp 5–20.

3. Guyatt GH, Keller JL, Jaeschke R, et al: The n-of-1 randomized control trial: Clinical usefulness. Our three-year experience. Ann Intern Med 112:293–299, 1990.

4. Guyatt G, Rennie D: Users' Guides to the Medical Literature: A Manual for Evidence-Based Clinical Practice. Chicago, American Medical Association, 2002.

5. Larson EB, Ellsworth AJ, Oas J: Randomized clinical trials in single patients during a 2-year period. JAMA 270:2708–2712, 1993.

6. Levine M, Haslam D, Walter S, et al: Harm. In Guyatt GH, Rennie D (eds): Users' Guides to the Medical Literature: A Manual for Evidence-Based Clinical Practice. Chicago, American Medical Association, 2002, pp 121–153.

7. Mahon J, Laupacis A, Donner A, Wood T: Randomised study of n of 1 trials versus standard practice. BMJ 312:1069–1074, 1996.

8. Millar AJ, Cywes S: Caustic strictures of the esophagus. In O'Neill JA, Rowe MI, Grosfeld JL, Coran AG (eds): Pediatric Surgery, 5th ed. St. Louis, Mosby, 1998, pp 969–979.

9. Sackett DL, Straus S, Richardson S, et al: Evidence-based Medicine: How to Practice and Teach EBM, 2nd ed. London, Churchill Livingstone, 2000.

INTRODUCTION TO BIOSTATISTIC CONCEPTS

Richard I. Wittman, MD, MPH, and Sue Kim, MD, MS

CHAPTER 9

1. **What is biostatistics?**
   Biostatistics provides a framework for the analysis of data. Through the application of statistic principles to the biologic sciences, biostatisticians (and others familiar with the collection, organization, analysis, and interpretation of data) are able to methodically distinguish between true differences among observations and random variations caused by chance alone.

2. **How is biostatistics useful?**
   From an application standpoint, knowledge of biostatistics and epidemiology permits one to make valid conclusions from data sets. Associations between risk factors and disease are determined with this information and, ultimately, are used to reduce illness and injury. Through the use of these methods, scientists and biostatisticians were able to demonstrate associations between benzene exposure and an increased risk of leukemia, and also between asbestos exposure and an increased risk of mesothelioma.

3. **What is the difference between nominal and ordinal variables?**
   - **Nominal (i.e., categorical) variables** represent data categorized by name alone, without consideration to order or magnitude of the variable. These data are not usually numeric. Examples include the following: blood type (A, B, AB, O), gender (female or male), eye color, and dichotomous (yes/no) events.
   - **Ordinal variables** can be considered as nominal variables classified into ordered or ranked categories, but not necessarily according to magnitude. Intervals (i.e., differences) among the categories may not be equal. Examples include the following: level of education completed (e.g., high school, college, or graduate), and questionnaire ranking (e.g., poor, fair, good, or excellent).

4. **Describe how interval, ratio, discrete, and continuous variables differ?**
   - **Interval variables** are similar to ordinal variables, but interval variables are spaced with equal intervals or distances; the zero point is not considered meaningful. An intelligence quotient (IQ) score would be an example.
   - **Ratio variables** are also categorized in ordered groups with equivalent intervals between the variables, but their zero point is meaningful. Body weight is an example.
   - **Discrete variables** represent data with an assigned order and magnitude but are restricted to whole numbers or integers; examples include money and the number of rooms in a hotel.
   - **Continuous variables** represent data capable of possessing any value in a given range, such as blood pressure, temperature, and weight.

5. **What are the different ways to describe these data types in chart form?**
   Nominal and ordinal data are best described and represented in *bar charts* and *pie graphs*. Discrete and continuous data are best displayed as *histograms* (which appear like a bar chart, but with the bars touching each other), *frequency polygons*, *scatter plots*, *box plots*, and *line graphs*.

6. **What is a measure of central tendency?**

The measures of central tendency—the mean, the median, and the mode—offer quick and concise specifics regarding the distribution of data and are a simple apparatus for communicating this pertinent data to others. In short, these measures provide information regarding the data composing the bulk of a distribution.

KEY POINTS: THREE MEASURES OF CENTRAL TENDENCY

1. Mean

2. Median

3. Mode

---

7. **How do I determine the value of the median?**

The median is used for ordinal, interval, ratio, discrete, and continuous data; it is defined as the 50th percentile of a set of measurements, the level below which half of the observations fall. For example, the median of the following five numbers (1, 1, 4, 9, 25) = 4. If there is an even number of variables being measured, the median represents the average of the two middle values.

The median is less affected by outliers (i.e., unusually high or low values) than the *mean*; in other words, it is a better measure of central tendency for skewed data. As such, it is considered the most robust measure of central tendency.

8. **How do the mean, median, and mode differ in their expression of central tendency?**

- The **mean** is used for interval and ratio data and is computed as the arithmetic mean (i.e., average) of the data. For example, the mean of the following five variables $(1, 1, 4, 9, 25) = \frac{40}{5} = 8$. The mean is more affected than the median by outliers.
- The **mode** is used for all types of data and represents the most frequently occurring observation. For example, the mode of the following five variables (1, 1, 4, 9, 25) = 1.
- The **median** is discussed in question 7.

9. **What is a measure of dispersion?**

Measures of dispersion describe the distribution or spread of the data. Used in conjunction with the measures of central tendency, they help to provide a more complete description of the data. Four commonly used measures of dispersion are the *range*, the *interquartile range*, the *variance*, and the *standard deviation*.

10. **What is the difference between range and interquartile range?**

- **Range** is the difference between the largest and the smallest value in the data distribution.
- **Interquartile range** describes the middle 50% of the observations (i.e., the data that fall in the 25th–75th percentiles).

11. **How do variance and standard deviation differ?**

- **Variance (s^2)** describes the amount of overall variability around the mean (in all directions) and is measured as the average of the squared distances between each variable and the mean. Mathematically, it is calculated as the following:

$$s^2 = \frac{1}{(n-1)} \sum_{i=1}^{n} (x_i - \bar{x})^2.$$

This will be discussed in more detail in later chapters.

- **Standard deviation (s)** is calculated as the positive square root of the variance: $(s = \sqrt{s^2})$.
  Because standard deviation describes the variability of the data in one direction only, it has the same units of measurement as the mean; hence, it is used more frequently than the variance to describe the breadth of the data.

12. **What is the Gaussian distribution? How does it relate to the empirical rule?**
   A Gaussian distribution is a *normal* or "bell-shaped" distribution of data which is symmetric around the mean; in this type of distribution, the *mean, median*, and *mode* all have the same value (Fig. 9-1). In such a distribution, the *empirical rule* states that roughly 68% of the data will be within one standard deviation of the mean (between the two inside lines, depicted below), roughly 95% of the distribution will be within two standard deviations of the mean (between the two out-side lines), and approximately 99.7% of the data will be within three standard deviations of the mean. To reiterate, in a normal or Gaussian distribution, the measures of central tendency are all equal and are located at the peak of distribution curve. (Also see Fig. 10-2.)

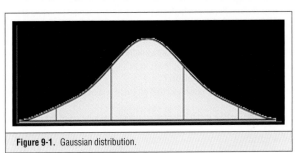

Figure 9-1. Gaussian distribution.

13. **Who was Gauss?**
   Karl Friedrich Gauss (1777–1855) was one of the foremost mathematicians of his time, advancing discoveries in number theory, algebra, geometry, probability, and other areas.

14. **What is Chebyshev's inequality?**
   When the distribution of data is not symmetric and cannot be described by a Gaussian distribution, it is still possible to generalize regarding data distribution or dispersion. In this situation, Chebyshev's inequality can be used as a conservative estimation of the *empirical rule* discussed above. It states that $\left[1 - \left(\frac{1}{k}\right)^2\right]$ of the data lie within k standard deviations of the mean. It can be very useful for application to skewed data sets.

15. **How do I determine in which direction the data are skewed?**
   A curve or distribution is *skewed* if the data are asymmetrically distributed. The data curve is termed to be skewed to the left (or negatively skewed) if the longer tail of the curve extends to the left and positively skews if the tail extends to the right. In such a curve, the mode is situated on the highest point on the curve, the mean is located toward the longer tail, and the median is situated between the mode and the mean, as depicted in Figure 9-2.

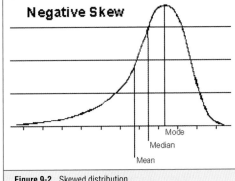

Figure 9-2. Skewed distribution.

KEY POINTS: FOUR MEASURES OF DISPERSION*

1. Range

2. Interquartile range

3. Variance

4. Standard deviation

*Similar logic applies when analyzing a curve (positively) skewed to the right.

16. **How can I tell if a data distribution exhibits kurtosis?**
    Kurtosis refers to the appearance of the peak of a curve, as well as to its tail, relative to a normal distribution. Data distributions with high kurtosis generally exhibit high and steep peaks near the mean, with wider tails; data with low kurtosis exhibit broader and flatter peaks than the normal distribution. A Gaussian distributed curve has zero skew and zero kurtosis. In a kurtotic distribution, the variance of the data remains unchanged.

17. **What is probability determination?**
    - **Probability (P)** refers to the likelihood that an event will or will not occur, based upon other factors.
    - **Probability determination** is the actual mathematic calculation of the likelihood of an event occurring.

18. **What is conditional probability?**
    Conditional probability reflects the likelihood that event A occurs, given that event B has occurred; in other words, the outcome of event A is dependent upon the occurrence and outcome of event B. This is notated as $P(B \mid A)$, or "the probability of event B occurring, given that A has already occurred." An example might be the probability of driving through two sequential green lights. The probability of driving successfully through the second green light requires that one was able to catch the first green light.

19. **What is an example of a mutually exclusive event?**
    Events are considered to be mutually exclusive if the occurrence of one event or outcome precludes the occurrence of the other outcome; in other words, mutually exclusive events cannot occur simultaneously. A common example is the "heads" or "tails" outcome after flipping a coin. In mutually exclusive events, the sum of the probabilities of the events is always less than or equal to 1. In contrast, events are determined to be independent if one event has no effect on the outcome of the other.

20. **In probability determination, what are the terms union, intersection, and complement?**
    - The **union** ($\cup$) of two events, A and B, is notated as $P(A \cup B)$. In the Venn diagram (Fig. 9-3), the union of A and B is represented by the entire area inside both circles, or A+B–C. The union represents the likelihood of the occurrence of event A alone, event B alone, and both events A and B simultaneously.
    - The **intersection** ($\cap$) of two events is defined as the event that is both A and B. The intersection of A and B is notated as $P(A \cap B)$; pictorially, this can be represented by area C in the Venn diagram (see Fig. 9-3).
    - The **complement** of an event A is "the event that is 'not A.'" Pictorially, it can be represented by the entire region outside of circle A. The complement is notated as A^c or $\overline{A}$.

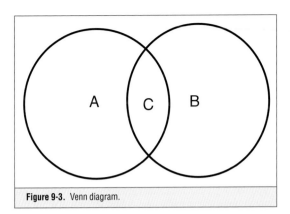

Figure 9-3. Venn diagram.

21. **What is the additive law of probability?**
    The additive law applies when events A and B cannot occur simultaneously, when they are mutually exclusive events. The additive law states that the probability of either event A or event B occurring is the probability of event A plus the probability of event B. This intuitively makes sense, for, if we were to flip a coin, the probability of either a "heads" (0.5) or a "tails" (0.5) would be equal to 1. The additive law in this case is notated as the following: $P(A \text{ or } B) = P(A) + P(B)$.

22. **Does the additive law apply when two events are *not* mutually exclusive?**
    No, the additive law does not apply. Instead, the probability of either event A or event B occurring is the probability of event A plus the probability of B, minus the probability that both events occur simultaneously—since if both occur at the same time, neither event A nor B can occur alone. This is notated as $P(A \text{ or } B) = P(A \cup B) = P(A) + P(B) - P(A \cap B)$, and describes the union operation previously discussed. The *additive law* for mutually exclusive events closely resembles this equation; when events are mutually exclusive, the probability (P) of both A and B occurring at the same time = 0, or $P(A \cap B) = 0$; substituted into the above equation, this yields the additive law, $P(A) + P(B)$.

KEY POINTS: DATA DISTRIBUTION IN A NORMAL GAUSSIAN DISTRIBUTION

1. Roughly 68% of the data fall within 1 standard deviation of the mean.

2. Roughly 95% of the data fall within 2 standard deviations of the mean.

3. Roughly 99.7% of the data fall within 3 standard deviations of the mean.

23. **What is the multiplicative law of probability?**
    The multiplicative law applies when event A and event B are conditionally dependent (and hence not mutually exclusive events). It states that the probability *(P)* that both events A and B will occur together is the probability of A times the probability of B, given that event A has already occurred. This is notated as the following: $P(A \text{ and } B) = P(A \cap B) = P(A) \times P(B|A)$.
    A transformation of this equation leads to the following: $P(B|A) = P \dfrac{(A \cap B)}{P(A)}$. This law will be discussed in more detail in a later chapter.

24. **Does the multiplicative law apply when two events are independent?**

    Not quite. If A and B are independent events (and hence neither mutually exclusive nor conditional events), the probability that *both events* will occur equals the probability of event A times the probability of event B. This is notated as $P(A \text{ and } B) = P(A) \times P(B)$. Given the same "heads" (0.5) and "tails" (0.5) example, the probability of exactly one "heads" and then exactly one "tails" on *two* successive coin flips would be 0.5×0.5, or 0.25.

    The multiplicative law is a special form of this equation, for when events A and B are independent the probability of event B occurring, given A has occurred, or $(P(B \mid A))$, equals $P(B)$; substitution of $P(B \mid A)$ for $P(B)$ into the above equation yields the multiplicative law (as described in question 23).

    $$P(A \text{ and } B) = P(A) \times P(B \mid A).$$

25. **What is statistic inference?**

    Statistic inference is the process of drawing conclusions regarding a population based upon studying only a portion of the members of that population. This process of inference (i.e., generalization), based upon a relative few, is most accurate when the subpopulation being studied is homogenous (i.e., uniform in character), when the subpopulation is truly representative (i.e., correctly reflects the larger group), and when the subpopulation is chosen randomly to eliminate sampling error or bias.

26. **How does one perform hypothesis testing?**

    Hypothesis testing is a way to perform statistic inference. It allows us to draw conclusions and make statements based upon the information obtained from the sample being analyzed. Most commonly in hypothesis testing, we assume that the mean (i.e., average) of the sample being studied is the same as the mean for the entire population from which the sample was drawn. We then attempt to prove or disprove this statement; for example, we may attempt to show that a new medication is superior to the standard treatment for a condition.

27. **What is meant by the null hypothesis?**

    In hypothesis testing, the null hypothesis states that there is no difference in population parameters among the groups being compared and that any observed differences are simply a result of random variation in the data rather than a result of actual disparity in the data itself. By convention, it is presumed that the null hypothesis is true (i.e., investigators assume the null hypothesis) at the outset of the study; the investigators then attempt to refute or reject this hypothesis through statistic analysis of the data.

28. **What is meant by the alternative hypothesis?**

    The alternative hypothesis serves as the opposing option to the null hypothesis. It contradicts the null hypothesis, stating that there is, in fact, a true difference (beyond that probable by random chance alone) in population parameters between or among the groups being compared.

29. **What does it mean for something to be statistically significant?**

    The difference between groups or data being compared is considered to be statistically significant when it exceeds an arbitrary cutoff level, which is designated by the investigator. This cutoff level is known as *alpha* (α) and is, by convention, often set at 0.05 or 5%; α represents the investigator's willingness to accept a 5% chance of failing to find a difference between the samples when, in fact, a true difference between the groups exists. Statistic significance does not indicate that the study itself is clinically significant; groups may exhibit substantial differences in measurements by statistic analysis, but these statistic differences may not translate into real-life differences between groups.

30. **What is the *p*-value?**

    The *p*-value is a numeric representation of the degree to which random variation alone could account for the differences observed between groups or data being compared. A study that finds a *p*-value of .05 asserts that there is a 5% chance of obtaining a result as extreme or more extreme than the actual observed or measured value by chance alone. The smaller the *p*-value, the stronger the evidence to dispute the null hypothesis; in other words, any difference observed in the study is more likely to be real, rather than due to chance alone.

31. **What is the relationship between the *p*-value and α?**
    When the *p*-value is less than the α cutoff, we say that the result is statistically significant. In the case of an α set at 0.05, a *p*-value <.001 is considered to be very strong evidence against the null hypothesis. A *p*-value >.10, however, is greater than α and represents weak evidence to dispute the null hypothesis, meaning that it is more likely that any observed or measured difference is due to random chance rather than an actual difference between groups.

KEY POINTS: HYPOTHESIS TESTING

1. Alpha (α): probability of making a type I error

2. Type I error: null rejection error (i.e., should not have rejected null)

3. Beta (β): probability of making a type II error

4. Type II error: null acceptance error (i.e., should not have failed to reject the accepted null)

5. Power = $1 - \beta$

32. **What is a type I error in hypothesis testing?**
    A type I error (i.e., rejection error or α-error) occurs when the null hypothesis is rejected (i.e., we say there is an actual difference between the groups or data) when, in fact, there is no true difference between the groups or data. Thus, a type I error can be considered a false-positive result.

33. **What is a type II error?**
    A type II error (i.e., an acceptance error or β-error) occurs when the null hypothesis is not rejected (i.e., the investigators say there is no difference between the groups or data) when, in reality, an actual difference exists. Thus, a type II error can be considered a false-negative result. There is a trade-off that exists between assigning the cutoffs for a type I error and for a type II error. (*See* Table 9-1.)

TABLE 9-1. HOW TO DETERMINE ERROR TYPE IN HYPOTHESIS TESTING

Outcome of Statistical Testing	True Population Data Results	
	Total Population Mean and Sampled Subpopulation Mean Are Equal	**Total Population Mean and Sampled Subpopulation Mean Are Different**
Do not reject null	Proper conclusion	Type II error (i.e., false negative, acceptance error, or ß-error)
Reject null	Type I error (i.e., false positive, rejection error, or α-error)	Proper conclusion

34. **What is the relationship between power and beta (β)?**

Power is defined as the probability of either correctly rejecting the null hypothesis when a true difference between groups does exist or correctly accepting (i.e., failing to reject) the null hypothesis when there is no actual difference between groups; thus, *power* is the probability of avoiding a type II error (i.e., not rejecting the null when it is false) and is equal to $1-\beta$. By convention, a power greater than or equal to 80% is considered acceptable.

35. **What are two ways to increase the power of a study?**

Although the power of a study is not under the control of the investigator, it is possible to increase the power of a study by *increasing the α-value*, leading to a decreased β and, hence, increased power. One can also increase power by *increasing the sample size* (i.e., the number of individuals or items involved in the study).

36. **How can biostatistics be applied to screening procedures to determine the likelihood of an individual having a disease?**

Screening tests are used to detect diseases in stages earlier than is possible by routine follow-up; therefore, detection must occur at times when intervention can alter the natural course of the disease and, ultimately, lead to improved quality or quantity of life for the affected individuals. It is important to consider that any intervention to prevent or treat a disease, when applied inappropriately, can lead to adverse consequences; thus, screening tests must correctly distinguish those who truly have the disease in question from those who do not. From a biostatistic standpoint, screening tests that possess both high sensitivity and high specificity are considered effective.

37. **What is meant by sensitivity and specificity?**

- **Sensitivity** is a measure of a test's ability to accurately identify disease when it is present. A test with a high sensitivity yields a high percentage of positive test results when disease is present (i.e., true positives) and produces few or no false negative results; thus, sensitivity is the probability of a test yielding a positive result when disease is present, which can be represented as $P(T^+ \mid D^+)$.
- **Specificity** is the probability of a negative test when disease is absent. A test with a high specificity tends to yield a negative test result when disease is absent (i.e., true negatives) and produces few or no false positive results. Specificity asks, "Given that disease is absent, what is the likelihood that a test will be negative?" It is represented as $P(T^- \mid D^-)$.

38. **What is meant by the predictive value of a test?**

- The **positive predictive value** (PPV) is similar to sensitivity, but instead of examining the probability of a positive test result when disease is present, it examines the probability of disease when the test is positive. It asks, "Given that the test is positive, what is the likelihood that disease is truly present?" PPV can be represented as $P(D^+ \mid T^+)$.
- The **negative predictive value** (NPV) of a test represents the probability that the disease is absent when there is a negative test. It asks, "Given that the test is negative, what is the likelihood that disease is truly absent?" NPV can be represented as $P(D^- \mid T^-)$.

39. **How do sensitivity and specificity differ from predictive value?**

As noted above, sensitivity and specificity refer to the likelihood of a positive or negative test result when disease is present or absent, respectively. The predictive value of a test refers to the likelihood of disease based upon the test result. Sensitivity and specificity are properties inherent to the test and do not vary with disease prevalence. Predictive values vary directly with the prevalence of the disease within the tested population.

40. **What is meant by a false-positive or false-negative test?**

- A **false-positive test** occurs when the test incorrectly reports disease presence when disease is, in fact, absent.
- A **false-negative test** occurs when the test incorrectly reports the absence of disease when disease is, in fact, present. (*See* Table 9-2.)

TABLE 9-2. GRAPHIC REPRESENTATION OF METHODS FOR OUTCOME ANALYSIS AFTER SCREENING FOR DISEASE

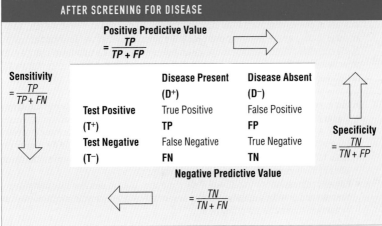

Positive Predictive Value
$$= \frac{TP}{TP + FP}$$

Sensitivity
$$= \frac{TP}{TP + FN}$$

	Disease Present (D⁺)	Disease Absent (D⁻)
Test Positive (T⁺)	True Positive **TP**	False Positive **FP**
Test Negative (T⁻)	False Negative **FN**	True Negative **TN**

Specificity
$$= \frac{TN}{TN + FP}$$

Negative Predictive Value
$$= \frac{TN}{TN + FN}$$

41. **What is a receiver operator curve (ROC)?**
The ROC is a graph that represents the relationship between sensitivity and specificity, with the "true positive rate" (i.e., sensitivity) appearing on the y-axis, and the "false positive rate" (1–specificity) appearing on the x-axis. This type of graph can help investigators assess the utility of a diagnostic test, for it can help determine the appropriate cutoff point for a screening test. In general, the point on the curve that lies closest to the left-hand top corner of the graph is taken as the point at which both sensitivity and specificity are maximized.

42. **What is a confidence interval?**
The mean of a sample population is only a point estimate of the mean for the entire population under study; although this sample mean may truly reflect the population mean, there is uncertainty in this value. Confidence intervals are constructs used to describe the range of values possible for this point estimate. The commonly used 95% confidence interval represents 95% confidence that the lower and upper limits of this interval include the true mean of the population being sampled. For example, if we randomly selected 100 samples from the population and determined 100 different confidence intervals for the means of these samples, 95 of the confidence intervals would include the true mean of the population, and 5 might not.

KEY POINTS: SCREENING

1. Sensitivity $= \frac{TP}{TP + FN}$ = true-positive rate = 1 – false-negative rate

2. Specificity $= \frac{TN}{TN + FP}$ = true-negative rate = 1 – false-positive rate

3. Negative predictive value $= \frac{TN}{TN + FN}$

4. Positive predictive value $= \frac{TP}{TP + FP}$

5. False negative rate $= \frac{FN}{FN + TP}$ = 1 – sensitivity = 100 – % sensitivity

6. False positive rate $= \frac{FP}{FP + TN}$ = 1 – specificity = 100 – % specificity

43. **What does it mean if two variables are correlated?**
Correlation between variables reflects the degree to which changes in one variable are related to changes in another variable. Variables can be correlated in a positive direction (i.e., an increase in one variable leads to an increase in the other) or a negative direction (i.e., an increase in one variable leads to a decrease in the other). Variables are described as being 100% correlated when a change in one variable always leads to a proportional change in the other variable. A Pearson correlation coefficient equal to +1 describes variables that are 100% correlated; a Pearson correlation coefficient of zero denotes variables with no correlation.

44. **What is regression? How do linear regression and logistic regression differ?**
   - **Linear regression** is a type of analysis used to describe the probability of outcome occurrence, a dependent variable, based upon the relationship between two or more independent *continuous random variables*; it is used to predict how changes in one (in the case of simple linear regression) or many (in the case of multiple linear regression) variables can affect the value of the dependent outcome of interest, represented as x.
   - **Logistic regression** is a variation of linear regression used to describe the relationship between two or more variables when the *dependent outcome variable is dichotomous* and the *independent variables are of any type.*

45. **What is survival analysis?**
Survival analysis aims to determine probabilities of "survival" for individuals from a designated starting time to a later point; this interval is called the **survival time**. The endpoint under study is referred to as a failure. Failure does not always signify death, but may also define outcomes such as the development of a particular disease or a disease relapse.

46. **Why is survival analysis distinct from other forms of regression?**
Survival analysis requires an approach that is different from logistic and linear regression for two reasons: (1) the data lack a normal distribution (i.e., the distribution of survival data tends to be skewed to the right) and (2) data censoring (i.e., there are incomplete observation times due to loss to follow-up or patient withdrawal from a study). Potential tools for analysis include life tables, the Kaplan-Meier method (i.e., the product-limit method), the log-rank test, and Cox regression.

WEBSITE

http://www.apps.nccd.cdc.gov/brfssdatasystems /estimates.asp

BIBLIOGRAPHY

1. Morton RF, Hebel JR, McCarter RJ: A Study Guide to Epidemiology and Biostatistics, 4th ed. Gaithersburg, Maryland, Aspen Publications, 1996.
2. Norman GR, Streiner DL: Biostatistics: The Bare Essentials, 2nd ed. Hamilton, Ontario, B.C. Decker, 2000.
3. Pagano M, Gauvreau K: Principles of Biostatistics, 2nd ed. Pacific Grove, CA, Duxbury Press, 2000.

CHAPTER 10

DESCRIBING AND SUMMARIZING DATA

Adam M. Brown, DO, and Robert J. Nordness, MD, MPH

1. **Define *variable*.**
   A variable is anything that can be measured and is observed to vary. Any measurement that is kept only at a single value cannot be a variable and is appropriately called a constant.

2. **How are data typically characterized?**
   Data are typically characterized as either quantitative or qualitative.

3. **What are quantitative data?**
   Data that are measured on a numeric or quantitative scale are considered quantitative. The information may be counted as discrete integer values or on a continuous scale. The ordinal, interval, and ratio scales are quantitative. A country's population, a person's shoe size, and a car's speed are all examples of quantitative information.

4. **Explain continuous variables.**
   Variables that can take on any value in a certain range or continuum are termed continuous variables. Time and distance are continuous, whereas gender, SAT scores, and "time rounded to the nearest second" are not. Quantitative variables that are not continuous are known as discrete variables. No measured variable is truly continuous; however, discrete variables measured with enough precision can often be considered continuous for practical purposes.

5. **Explain discrete variables.**
   Variables that can only take on a finite number of values are called discrete variables. All qualitative variables are discrete. Some quantitative variables are discrete, such as "performance rated as 1, 2, 3, 4, or 5," and "temperature rounded to the nearest degree." Discrete variables are values equal to integers; another example is the number of fractures present in a trauma patient.

   Sometimes a variable that takes on enough discrete values can be considered to be continuous for practical purposes. One example is time rounded to the nearest millisecond. Variables that can take on an infinite number of possible values are called continuous variables.

6. **What are qualitative data?**
   Also termed categoric data, qualitative data are variables with no natural sense of ordering. For instance, hair color (e.g., black, brown, gray, red, or yellow) is qualitative information, as is name (e.g., Adam, Becky, Christina, or Dave). Qualitative factors can be coded to appear numeric, but their numbers are meaningless from a quantitative standpoint, as in male = 1, female = 2.

7. **Are variables quantitative or qualitative?**
   Variables can be either quantitative or qualitative, and the type of variable described is a significant factor in subsequent statistic analysis.

8. **What makes a variable independent?**
   An independent variable can be conceptualized as a hypothesized cause or influence on a dependent variable; typically, the outcome of interest. An independent variable can be a factor

that you control, like a treatment, or an exposure that is not controlled, or perhaps a demographic factor like age or gender.

9. **What are dependent variables?**

The dependent variable is the outcome being investigated. A study attempts to determine whether an association exists between the potential risk factors (i.e., independent variables) and the dependent variable of interest.

10. **Describe the relationship between independent variables and dependent variables.**

The concept of independent and dependent variables is analogous to that seen in introductory algebra. One or more independent variables undergo some sort of arithmetic operation, often with the introduction of constants, to determine the value of the dependent variable. In the equation $F = 1.8 \times C + 32$, C is the *independent variable* and F the *dependent variable* because changes in F depend on changes in C. If the equation were written $C = (F - 32) / 1.8$, then C would be the dependent variable and F the independent variable. This example also illustrates that a property or characteristic may be thought of as a risk factor in some contexts and as an outcome in others.

11. **What are some commonly used scales of measurement?**

The scales of measurement can be divided into four categories:

- Nominal scale
- Ordinal scale
- Interval scale
- Ratio scale

12. **Describe the nominal scale.**

Nominal scales are used to group qualitative data into arbitrary categories with no inherent order. A good example is race/ethnicity, with the following values: 1 = white, 2 = Hispanic, 3 = American Indian, 4 = black, 5 = other. Note that the assigned numeric values and the order of the categories are arbitrary. Certain statistic concepts are meaningless for nominal data. For example, it would be silly to calculate the mean and standard deviation for race/ethnicity.

13. **Describe the ordinal scale.**

Ordinal scales rank categorical data in a manner that has a logical ordering to the categories. A good example is the Likert scale, which you see on many surveys: 1 = strongly disagree; 2 = disagree; 3 = neutral; 4 = agree; 5 = strongly agree. Ordinal scales show relative ranking, but one cannot make any assumptions about the degree of difference between two values.

14. **Describe the interval scale**

The interval scale is similar to the ordinal scale in that there is a sequential ranking of the values assigned. An interval scale also has the property of having a meaningful (i.e., an equal) difference between the successive values in the scale. The Fahrenheit and Celsius temperature scales are classic examples of interval scales. The difference between 70° and 80°F is exactly the same as the difference between 30° and 40°F.

15. **How is the ratio scale different from the interval scale?**

The ratio scale is similar to the interval scale in that there is a meaningful ranking of the values in the scale, and also in that the difference between any two values is both meaningful and of equal magnitude. What makes the ratio scale unique is that the zero value is meaningful. For example, a weight of zero means the absence of matter, whereas the temperature of 0°F is totally arbitrary.

16. **What is the significance of a meaningful zero value in the ratio scale?**
    The implication of a meaningful zero value is that the ratio of two values is also meaningful. For example, consider again weight, measured on a ratio scale. An object that weighs 10 lb is twice as heavy as something that weighs 5 lb. We cannot, however, claim that an object with a temperature of 10°F is twice as warm as that object at 5°F, as the zero value on the Fahrenheit scale is arbitrary.

KEY POINTS: VARIABLES AND SCALES OF MEASUREMENT

1. Variables take on various values.

2. Independent variables are used to estimate values for dependent variables.

3. Nominal scales are used to arbitrarily group qualitative data.

4. Ordinal scales show rank but give no information about the distance between values.

5. Interval scales have meaningful rank and spacing between values

6. Ratio scales have a meaningful zero, which gives meaning to the ratio of two values.

17. **What general measures are used to describe frequency distributions for quantitative data?**
    Measures of central tendency and measures of dispersion. Measures of central tendency describe a typical value of the distribution, whereas measures of dispersion give an idea of the spread of the values about the central measure.

18. **What are most commonly used measures of central tendency?**
    The mean, the median, and the mode.

19. **What is the mean value of a frequency distribution?**
    The mean is simply the arithmetic average of all the items in a sample. To compute a sample mean, add up all the sample values and divide by the size of the sample. For example, the cotinine values for seven smokers are: 73, 58, 67, 93, 33, 18, and 147. If you added these values you would get a sum of 489. Divide that sum by 7 to get a mean of 69.9.

$$\bar{x} = \frac{\sum_{i=1}^{n} x_i}{n} = (73 + 58 + 67 + 93 + 33 + 18 + 147)/7 = 69.9$$

20. **What is the median value?**
    The median is the middle value of an ordered frequency distribution, so that roughly half of the data are smaller and roughly half of the data are larger.

21. **How do you calculate the median value of a frequency distribution?**
    There are two formulas for the computation of the median, depending on whether the size of your sample is even or odd. In both cases, sort the data from smallest to largest.
    - If n (i.e., the number of observations in your sample) is **odd**, select the $(n + 1)/2$ observation. For example, consider these five cholesterol readings, measured in mg/dl: 128, 168, 188, 202, and 244. There are five values in the sample, so the $(n + 1)/2$ value is the third value (188) and the median.
    - If n is **even**, select halfway between the $n/2$ and $(n/2) + 1$ observation. In another sample of adults, the cholesterol values, in mg/dl, are: 164, 186, 222, 230, 272, and 288. For these data there are an even number of observations (n = 6). So we would select

halfway between the third observation (222) and the fourth observation (230). Thus, the median is (222 + 230)/2 = 226. Note that the median value in this set is not an actual value for any subject in the sample.

22. **Which is a more stable indicator of central tendency, the median or the mean?**
The median is a more stable indicator of central tendency. For example, 10 students scored the following results on a pop quiz in statistics: 41, 42, 42, 43, 44, 46, 48, 48, 50, and 98. The median value here is 45 and represents a typical (although not an actual) value in this sample. The mean, on the other hand, is 50.2, a score greater than 90% of the sample.

23. **What is the mode?**
The mode is simply the most commonly occurring value in a frequency distribution. The highest peak on a frequency represents the mode. A distribution may have any number of modes. Distributions with one mode are termed *unimodal*, those with two are termed *bimodal*, and so on.

KEY POINTS: CENTRAL TENDENCY

1. Mean, median, and mode are measures of central tendency.

2. The mean is simply the arithmetic average of the observed values.

3. The median divides the distribution into two equal groups.

4. The mode is the most commonly observed value in the distribution.

5. There may be more than one mode in any given data set.

6. The mean is affected more by extreme values than is the median.

24. **What is a skewed distribution?**
A distribution that is unbalanced by extreme scores at or near one end is said to be a skewed distribution. In graphic form, skewed distributions are labeled according to the direction of the tail; that is, when the tail goes to the left, the curve is negatively skewed; when the tail goes to the right, it is positively skewed. Distributions with positive skew are more common than distributions with negative skew. Figure 10-1 shows three separate types of skew: curve A is positively skewed or

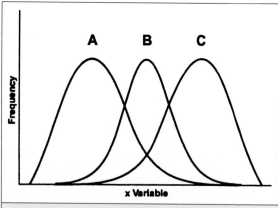

Figure 10-1. Effect of skewing on the mean, median, and mode. (From Centers for Disease Control and Prevention: Principles of Epidemiology, 2nd ed. Atlanta, U.S. Department of Health and Human Services, Public Health Service, Centers for Disease Control and Prevention, Epidemiology Program Office, Public Health Practice Program,1992.)

skewed to the right, curve B is symmetric and has no skew, whereas curve C is negatively skewed or skewed to the left. As a rule, the mean is larger than the median in positively skewed distributions and less than the median in negatively skewed distributions, as explained previously.

25. **Describe a real-world example of a skewed distribution.**

One example of skew is the distribution of income. Most people make under $40,000 per year, but some make quite a bit more, with a small number making many millions of dollars per year. The positive tail, therefore, extends outward quite a long way, whereas the negative tail stops at zero.

26. **What is the relationship among mean, median, and mode in a symmetric frequency distribution?**

In a symmetric frequency distribution, the mean and median are identical. In addition, if the distribution is both symmetric and unimodal, the mode is also equal to the mean and median. The curve on the left in Figure 10-2 shows a symmetric unimodal frequency distribution in which the mean, median, and mode are equal.

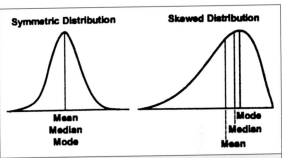

Figure 10-2. Areas under the normal curve that lie between 1, 2, and 3 standard deviations on each side of the mean. (From Centers for Disease Control and Prevention: Principles of Epidemiology, 2nd ed. Atlanta, U.S. Department of Health and Human Services, Public Health Service, Centers for Disease Control and Prevention, Epidemiology Program Office, Public Health Practice Program,1992.)

27. **What is the relationship between mean and median in skewed distributions?**

In skewed distributions, the extreme values will affect the mean to a larger degree than they will the median. The mean will "chase the tail" of skewed distributions, whereas the median will tend to stay home. These concepts are illustrated above. The negatively skewed curve on the right in Figure 10-2 illustrates the relationship of the mean, median, and mode when the distribution is skewed.

28. **What are the measures of dispersion commonly used in biostatistics?**

The most common measures of dispersion are the range, the standard deviation, and the variance.

29. **What is the range of a frequency distribution?**

The range (R) is the measurement of the width of the entire distribution and is found simply by calculating the difference between the highest and lowest scores. For example, if the highest score in an intelligence quotient (IQ) distribution is 160 and the lowest is 80, the R = 80, the difference between the highest and lowest scores. Based upon only theses two scores, the range gives no information about the distribution of the scores between these values.

30. **How are quantiles useful in describing frequency distributions?**

Quantiles divide frequency distributions into equal, ordered subgroups, giving more information about the data distribution than the range, which relies only on the highest and lowest values.

The most commonly used quantile is the quartile, which divides the data into four equally sized groups. Deciles divide the data into ten equal groups. We are all accustomed to the percentile, a system often used in describing rank in standardized test; for instance, a score in the 95th percentile indicates a superior performance to 95% of all those taking the exam.

31. **What is the interquartile range?**
As explained above, quartiles divide a distribution into quarters. The interquartile range is the difference between the first and third quartiles, or, in other words, it is the range of the middle 50% of the data. By definition, 25% of the values will be below those found in the interquartile range and 25% of the values will be greater.

32. **What is a standard deviation?**
The standard deviation is the most widely used measure of the spread of data about their mean. The larger the standard deviation, the more spread out the distribution of the data about the mean.

33. **How is the standard deviation of a sample calculated?**
The formula for the standard deviation is given below, where SD = standard deviation, $\sum$ = summation of, x = individual score, $\bar{x}$ (called "x-bar") = mean of all scores, and n = sample size (i.e., number of scores).

$$SD = \sqrt{\frac{\sum (x - \bar{x})^2}{n - 1}}$$

34. **Give an example problem calculating the standard deviation of a sample.**
Consider the following test scores from a college physics course in which seven students were present on test day: 76, 80, 84, 85, 88, 90, and 92. A quick glance at the data may give us a feel that the mean will be in the mid-80s. Calculation of the mean yields 85.0, which is consistent with our ballpark estimate. To calculate the standard deviation, we must subtract the mean from each individual value, square this difference, and then add all of the terms; this sum is know as the total sum of the squares (TSS):

$$TSS = \sum (X - mean)^2$$

$$\text{Where the } mean = \sum \frac{X}{n}$$

(n = the total number of subjects in the experiment)

$$(76-85)^2 + (80-85)^2 + (84-85)^2 + (85-85)^2 + (88-85)^2 + (90-85)^2 + (92-85)^2 = TSS = 190.$$

The TSS is now divided by n−1 (which is 6) to yield a term known as the variance:

$$Variance = \frac{TSS}{(n - 1)} = 31.67$$

The square root of this value is equal to the standard deviation, $SD = \sqrt{31.67} = 5.63$

35. **What is the variance?**
The variance is the measurement of the variation among all the subjects in an experiment. As illustrated in the calculation of standard deviation in the previous problem, the variance is simply the square of the standard deviation. Like standard deviation, the variance is a measure of the dispersion of the data set from the mean value. The variance is equal to the summation of the squared differences between each value and the mean, divided by the number of values in the data set, less one:

$$Variance = \frac{TSS}{(n - 1)}$$

$$Variance = (SD)^2$$

36. **In a normal distribution, how does the standard deviation help us to estimate expected values?**

Figure 10-3 illustrates the frequency distribution in a normal distribution in relation to the standard deviation. Overall, approximately 68% of the values should fall between two standard deviations from the mean (i.e., one SD above and one SD below the mean value). Over 95% of the values should fall between two standard deviations in either direction from the mean, and approximately 99% of the values should fall within three standard deviations from the mean. These values serve as useful ballpark estimators whenever a frequency distribution can reasonably be considered a normal distribution.

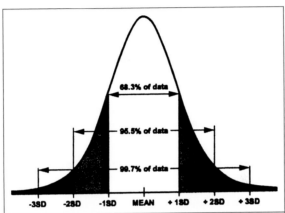

Figure 10-3. Three curves with different skewing. (From Centers for Disease Control and Prevention: Principles of Epidemiology, 2nd ed. Atlanta, U.S. Department of Health and Human Services, Public Health Service, Centers for Disease Control and Prevention, Epidemiology Program Office, Public Health Practice Program, 1992.)

37. **Describe the coefficient of variation.**

The coefficient of variation is a measure of the variability of the values in a sample, relative to the value of the mean. Mathematically, it is simply the ratio of standard deviation to the mean. Of note, the coefficient of variation is truly meaningful only for values measured on a ratio scale.

KEY POINTS: DISPERSION

1. Range, standard deviation, and variance are common measures of dispersion.

2. The range is simply the difference between the lowest and highest value, giving the width of the distribution but nothing else.

3. Standard deviation is the most commonly used measure of dispersion.

4. In a normal distribution, 68% of the values will fall between one standard deviation above and one standard deviation below the mean value.

5. Variance is simply the standard deviation squared.

38. **Define standard error of the mean (SEM).**
The standard error of the mean is simply an estimate of the accuracy of a sample mean in describing the mean of the population from which it was derived. If one took many samples from a given population, it is expected that the means would be slightly different, both from each other and from the true population mean. The standard error of the mean is simply an estimate of the standard deviation of a group of sample means around the population mean.

39. **How is the SEM calculated?**
The SEM is calculated very simply by dividing the standard deviation from a single sample by the square root of the number of observations in that sample.

$$SEM = \frac{SD}{\sqrt{n}}$$

40. **What is the use of the SEM?**
The SEM is used to construct confidence intervals around a sample mean. The smaller the SEM, the more confidence one has that the sample mean is truly representative of the population.

41. **Define measurement error.**
Measurement error is the variation in the measurement of observations that is attributable to the measuring process itself. Measurement variation is a term often used as a synonym for measurement error.

42. **Name the two types of measurement error that may be committed.**
Measurement error consists of systematic and random error.

43. **What is random measurement error?**
Random errors increase the dispersion and are equally likely to fall on either side of the true value. Random errors are considered to occur by chance and thus are not predictable. All data sampling is subject to random error. As the number of measurements in a sample increases, the discrepancy caused by random error will decrease and the summation of random error will tend toward zero.

44. **What is systematic measurement error?**
Systematic measurement error, also known as bias, is caused by a consistent fault in some aspect of the measurement process that causes the values to center around a value other than the true value. Increasing the number of observations has no effect on systematic error.

45. **What is precision?**
Precision is lack of random error, causing a close grouping in repeated measurements.

46. **What is validity?**
Validity is the lack of systematic error (i.e., bias) leading to measured values approaching the true value.

47. **What is a rate?**
In statistic terms, a rate is a measure of the frequency of an occurrence over some time interval. In epidemiology, demography, and vital statistics, a rate is an expression of the frequency with which an event occurs in a defined population in a specified period of time. Rates are ratios, calculated by dividing a numerator (e.g., the number of deaths or newly occurring cases of a disease in a given period) by a denominator (e.g., the average population during that period).

48. **What is a proportion?**

A proportion is a type of ratio in which the numerator is included in the denominator, which represents the entire sample. By definition, a proportion must have a value between 0 and 1. Because numerator and denominator have the same dimension, a proportion is a dimensionless quantity.

KEY POINTS: ERRORS

1. The standard error of the mean (SEM) is used to estimate the difference of a sample mean from that of the parent population.

2. Measurement errors are categorized as random or systematic errors.

3. Random errors create dispersion.

4. The effect of random error decreases as the number of observations increases.

5. Systematic error is also known as bias.

6. Systematic error is a consistent measurement error that centers observations at a value other than the true value.

49. **Provide an example of a proportion.**

Twenty students took a biostatistics quiz, and 15 of them passed. The proportion who failed = 5 students failed out of 20 students taking the test = 5/20 = 0.25. Proportions are often converted to percentages for convenience; one would say that 25% of the students who took the test failed.

WEBSITES

1. http://www.zebu.uoregon.edu/1999/es202/l16.html

2. http://www-phm.umds.ac.uk/teaching/ClinEpid/default.htm

3. http://www.consort-statement.org

4. http://www.psych.rice.edu/online_stat/glossary/skew.html

5. http://www.davidmlane.com/hyperstat/A92403.html

6. http://www.davidmlane.com/hyperstat/A11284.html

7. http://www.cs.umd.edu/~mstark/exp101/expvars.html

8. http://www.tufts.edu/~gdallal/LHSP.htm

BIBLIOGRAPHY

1. Bland JM, Altman DG: Statistics notes: Measurement error and correlation coefficients. BMJ 313:41–42, 1996.

2. Centers for Disease Control and Prevention: Principles of Epidemiology, 2nd ed. Atlanta, U.S. Department of Health and Human Services, Public Health Service, Centers for Disease Control and Prevention, Epidemiology Program Office, Public Health Practice Program,1992.

3. Devereaux PJ, Manns BJ, Ghali WA, et al: Physician interpretations and textbook definitions of blinding terminology in randomized controlled trials. JAMA 285:2000–2003, 2001.

4. Jekel JF, Katz DL, Elmore JG: Epidemiology, Biostatistics, and Preventive Medicine, 2nd ed. Philadelphia, W.B. Saunders, 2001.

5. Last JM (ed): A Dictionary of Epidemiology, 4th ed. Oxford, Oxford University Press, 2001.

6. Rothman KJ: Epidemiology: An Introduction. Oxford, Oxford University Press, 2002.

CHAPTER 11

FREQUENCY AND PROBABILITY DISTRIBUTIONS

Robert W. Perkins, MD, MPH

FREQUENCY DISTRIBUTIONS

1. **What is a frequency distribution?**

   A frequency distribution illustrates how often different data categories appear within a data sample. This information is presented in a variety of different formats, from simple tables to three-dimensional graphs and plots. Tabular data are useful when there are large numbers of variables to display. It also works well if you want to present data together that are significantly different in scale. For example, cumulative frequency on the x-axis always increases from zero to 100%, regardless of the category frequency on the y-axis. Such variation may make a graph unreadable when these data are plotted together. Presenting the same data in a table avoids this problem of scale.

2. **What is the difference between discrete and continuous data?**

   Discrete data have a circumscribed set of possible values. Continuous data are open ended with an infinite set of possible values. The presence of a meaningful distance between values is also helpful in separating data types. Consider the difference between letters and numbers. There is a meaningful distance between 2 and 3, and this distance is the same between any other pair of adjacent numbers. There is, however, no absolutely quantifiable distance between K and L. The concept of "distance" between letters is meaningless. For both of the above reasons, alphabets are discrete data sets and numbers are continuous.

3. **Describe the two types of discrete data and give examples of each.**

   - **Nominal data** consist of named categories with no defined relationship to any other category and no inherent order. Color names, for example, do not inherently define distance or value from one color to another, and they do not define any order among them. Red is not bigger than blue or farther from blue than purple is from orange. Those of you who are more astronomically minded may protest that colors do have order and meaningful distance, given their relative position in the visible light spectrum. However, this is really just the arbitrary application of discrete labels (i.e., color names) to a continuous property of light, the electromagnetic wavelength.

   - **Ordinal data** consist of named categories that, though lacking meaningful distance between them, do have established order among them. Letter grades in school illustrate how ordinal data tell you which category comes first, but tell you nothing about the relative distance among them. (For example, A's are better than D's, but the difference between an A and a B may not be the same as between a D and an F.)

4. **Answer question 3 again, this time for continuous data.**

   - **Interval data:** Celsius temperature is an example of interval data. One degree of difference in Celsius temperature is a quantifiable change that is preserved across the range of possible values. For example, 5°C is the same "distance" from 4°C degrees as 120°C is from 121°C. However, 100°C is not twice as hot as 50°C in terms of energy. This is because the zero point for Celsius temperature is arbitrarily set at the freezing point of water. Interval data have meaningful unit distance, but the ratio between values is not a meaningful quantity.

- **Ratio data:** Kelvin degrees are an example of ratio data. Kelvin degrees have order, meaningful distance, and a meaningful zero—absolute zero, to be precise. If we convert the relationship between 100°C and 50°C to Kelvin, we see that 373K / 323K = 1.15. So, with respect to absolute zero, 100°C is only about 15% hotter (or has only 15% more energy) than 50°C. The ratio between measurements in degrees Kelvin is a meaningful quantity which describes a truer relationship between states than do degrees Celsius.

As you can see, pinning down the exact difference between ratio and interval data is not always straightforward. Many types of data are often not exactly one or the other. This is generally not as critical to analysis as is the distinction between the "super-categories" of discrete and continuous data.

5. **How does the data type affect how distributions are presented?**
For discrete data (i.e., nominal and ordinal data), each category or class is plotted against the frequency with which that category occurs in the sample. For continuous data (i.e., interval and ratio data), every single data point is technically in its own category. Graphing the frequency of every individual data point (for all but very small data sets) results in cluttered graphs that do not convey much useful information.

6. **How can continuous data be presented more clearly?**
This type of data should first be grouped into ranges and then plotted according to the frequency with which data in each range appear in the sample. See Figure 11-1 for an example of a continuous data distribution.

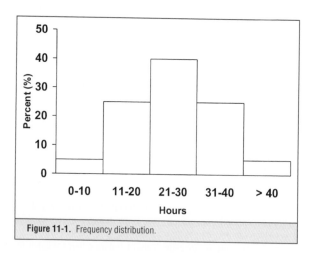

Figure 11-1. Frequency distribution.

7. **Describe three common uses for frequency distributions.**
- Frequency distributions are often used to present the results of analyzed data. Properly formatted, they convey a great deal of information in a simple, compact figure.
- They are particularly useful in the very earliest analysis of collected data. Plotting the raw data distribution often identifies outliers (i.e., abnormal highs or lows), missing data, and problems with biased data collection.
- A frequency distribution is also important in formulating a statistical analysis strategy, because some statistical tests require that the data be normally distributed.

8. **Name three values commonly used to characterize the central tendency of a data set.**
   - **Mean:** the sum of the values of the data points, divided by the number of values.
   - **Median:** the value of the middle data point, after the data have been sorted.
   - **Mode:** the most frequently occurring value.

9. **What term best describes the central tendency of interval and ratio data?**
   The best descriptor of central tendency depends on the type of data in the distribution. The mean is most often used to describe the central tendency of interval and ratio data. This calculation depends on meaningful distance among values and thus cannot be used for ordinal and nominal data. Letter grades are a good example. You cannot take two As, four Bs, one C, and one D, add them together, and divide by eight to get an average grade. However, if you assign an interval or ratio value to each grade (e.g., four point grade systems, in which A=4, B=3, etc.), then calculation of a mean grade is possible.

   If this bothers you, congratulations! You have clearly been paying attention. Because you started out with discrete data, there is an element of artificiality introduced by converting to a continuous grading scale and computing a mean from it. The mean calculation assumes a meaningful unit distance, which you never had to begin with. Not that this has ever been of much concern to any university registrar.

10. **How is central tendency measured for ordinal and nominal data?**
    Ordinal data, though they do not have meaningful distance between values, still have meaningful order. Consequently, the category with the middle, or median, value among the ordered categories describes the central value around which the data are distributed. Describing the central tendency of nominal data is limited to the mode. Because there is no meaningful distance among categories, and no order with which to determine the middle value, the most frequently occurring category (i.e., the mode) is the only way to express central tendency. Of course, there is nothing "central" at all about this number, because the categories of nominal data can be ordered any way you wish.

11. **What are measures of dispersion, and what is the best measure for each data type?**
    Measures of dispersion tell you, given a central tendency, how closely the rest of the data fall about that central value. Consequently, there is no measure of dispersion for the mode when used to describe nominal data. (Again, there is nothing "central" about this value.) For all other data types, the interquartile range (i.e., middle 50% of the data) best describes the dispersion about the mode. When the median is used to describe central tendency, dispersion is most commonly characterized by the range. The range is calculated by subtracting the lowest value from the highest, and is reported as a single number. For example, given the following data set (2, 3, 6, 9, 10, 22, 23), the range would be reported as 21, not 23–2. The standard deviation is the measure of dispersion most commonly used for interval and ratio data.

12. **How is the standard deviation computed?**
    First, compute the mean for the data. Then, for each measurement, compute the difference between the measurement and the mean. This will give you a column of data, both positive and negative, that represent the distance of each value from the mean. If you added them all together with the intent of computing an "average deviation," they would equal zero and would give you no good information about the average distance of your data from the mean.

13. **So how do you preserve the information on each deviation from the mean?**
    You square each result before adding them together, which removes all the negative numbers. Dividing the sum of these values by the total number of data points gives you an average distance from the mean, in squared units, known as the variance. Since squared units are not very meaningful, the square root of the variance is taken to restore the original units. This is the

standard deviation, given by $SD = \sqrt{\frac{\Sigma(X - \overline{X})^2}{N}}$, where X is the data value, $\overline{X}$ is the mean, and N is the number of data points. The formula for the variance (s^2) consists of everything under the square root sign. The formula above is used for calculation of the standard deviation of a population. More often in biostatistics, one is analyzing data from a sample of the population, in which case the correct formula for standard deviation of a sample is given by

$SD = \sqrt{\frac{\Sigma(X - \overline{X})^2}{n - 1}}$. Standard deviation is defined as the square root of the variance; therefore,

variance = (standard deviation)^2.

14. **Name three terms that are used to describe the shape of frequency distributions.**

Modality, skew, and kurtosis. "Modality," as used here, is a conventional term rather than a true property of a distribution. As described above, the mode refers to the most frequently occurring category. In a graph, it will be the peak category, and all the others will go down from there. Data sets with only one "most frequent" category result in a unimodal distribution; that is, a single peak category. If the data have two or more categories with notably higher frequencies, the distribution is bimodal, or trimodal, etc. This terminology is often used with interval and ratio data to describe distributions with multiple peaks, even though the mode is rarely used to describe these types of data. Figure 11-2 shows an example of a bimodal distribution.

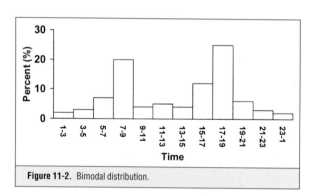

Figure 11-2. Bimodal distribution.

15. **What is skew? How does it affect the shape of the distribution?**

Skew refers to the symmetry of the data distribution. A distribution with no skew will be symmetric about the central value and will have a fairly equal distribution of decreasing values on either side. The distribution is said to be skewed to the right when the center of the data is shifted to the left, leaving a rightward tail of comparatively low-frequency, high-magnitude values. By convention, skew is referred to as right or left based on the direction of the tail (Fig. 11-3).

16. **Answer the same question as above for kurtosis.**

Kurtosis refers to how rapidly the frequency among the categories changes as you move away from the central value. If the frequency of each category drops off quickly as you move away, the distribution appears taller, narrower, and with less distribution in the tails (i.e., the distribution is leptokurtic). If the frequencies do not decrease quickly away from the central value, the distribution is flatter, wider, and has more values in the tails (i.e., the distribution is platykurtic).

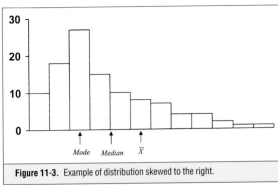

Figure 11-3. Example of distribution skewed to the right.

17. How are measures of central tendency and dispersion related to kurtosis?
Kurtosis is also related to the frequency (i.e., y-axis) of the central value. Consequently, varying degrees of kurtosis may reflect differences in the frequency of the central value, but they do not necessarily change the magnitude (i.e., x-axis) of the central value. Because kurtosis describes the width of a distribution about the middle value, it *will* be affected by varying degrees of dispersion.

18. How does skew affect these same measures?
Skew is the result of low-frequency categories with abnormally high or low values. By definition, low-frequency categories should not change the mode. Similarly, the median is relatively resistant to change from a few extreme value categories. It changes more than the mode because the middle value shifts somewhat when new categories are added at the extremes of the distribution. The calculation of the mean gives equal weight to outliers and central data alike, so it can change significantly with the addition of even a few extreme values. Figure 11-3 shows an example of the changes to mean, median, and mode in a skewed distribution.

19. How do extreme values affect distribution around the central values?
Extreme values can also influence the measures of dispersion. The range is defined by the extreme values and can be significantly changed with skewed data. The standard deviation weighs the deviation of each category from the mean equally, so low-frequency categories in the extremes do affect it, but not overwhelmingly. Because the interquartile range represents the middle 50% of the data, it is least affected by skew.

20. What is a normal distribution?
The normal (i.e., Gaussian) distribution is a mathematically defined shape that is symmetric about a mean of zero, has a skew and kurtosis of zero, and a median and mode that are both equal to the mean. It is a theoretical distribution, so the high and low values in the tails approach, but never reach, zero.

21. What is it good for?
Many processes of interest to researchers occur in approximately normal distributions. A mathematically normal distribution can simplify calculations when it is used to infer statistical properties from the near-normal real data. Means from repeated sampling of a given population tend to be normally distributed—a phenomenon described as the central limit theorem, but more on that later—and many statistical tests used to analyze sample data rely on the assumption of an approximately normal distribution.

22. **The normal distribution can be used to infer the properties of what two broad categories of data?**

The normal distribution can be used to infer the properties of both sample and population data. *Sample data* refers to a subset of data collected out of a given population. It would be the distribution of answers you got if you asked a sample of 100 motorcycle owners how much money they had spent on their bikes that year. The population distribution results from collecting that same data from *every* motorcycle owner over the same period.

23. **Why are sample data used instead of the population data?**

Sample data, by definition, are relatively obtainable. Population data are generally not. Population data will often evolve and change before you can collect the entire data set. This will introduce error if the 100,000th data point is recorded in a different state or point in time than the first. Sample data are designed to be of sufficient size to give meaningful information about the population they come from, yet still be recorded before too much change occurs. Finally, with all but the smallest populations, the real-world costs of collecting population data are generally prohibitive.

24. **Describe the relationship between the area under the curve of a distribution and the percent of data that fall in that range.**

In any distribution, the area under the curve bounded by two limits is proportional to the percent of the data in the sample that fall between those limits. If you want to know what proportion of your sample falls between two particular values, this is a convenient property. Figure 11-4 illustrates the area under the curve between two arbitrary values. This area would be proportional to the percent of all the data sampled that fall between 12 and 16.

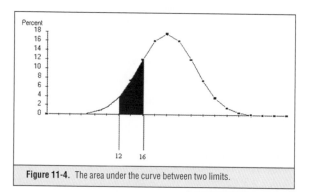

Figure 11-4. The area under the curve between two limits.

25. **How do you calculate the exact proportion from the distribution?**

Unfortunately, before the wide availability of computer software, calculating an area for every possible combination of limits was complicated and impractical, and the calculation had to be redone for each new data set. The area under the normal curve was instead calculated between the mean and several increasingly distant values from that mean. The results were compiled into large tables and users could then extrapolate the values of interest from between the tabulated values.

26. **How does the normal distribution help solve this problem?**

Statisticians realized that if sample data were approximately normally distributed, you could use a table made for the normal distribution to calculate the area under the curve for the sample distribution. Figure 11-5 shows a sample distribution in which the mean is 10 and the sample standard deviation is 2. To figure the area under the curve between 8 and 10, you simply need to find

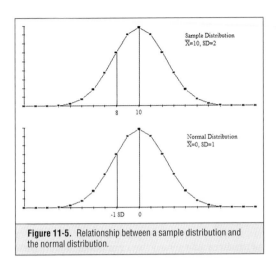

Figure 11-5. Relationship between a sample distribution and the normal distribution.

out which value in the normal distribution has the same relative distance from zero as the value of interest (i.e., 8) does from the mean in your sample distribution (i.e., 10).

27. How can values from real data be compared to a "unit-less" theoretic distribution?

By computing the distance of the sample value of interest from the sample mean in standard deviation units. This calculation, known as the zee score, is given by $z = \left(\dfrac{X - \bar{X}}{s}\right)$, where X is the sample data point, $\bar{X}$ is the sample mean, and s is the sample standard deviation. In Figure 5, the zee score is $\left(\dfrac{8 - 10}{2}\right)$, or −1. If the sample is normally distributed, the percent of data falling between 8 and 10 in the sample is proportional to the area under the curve between 0 and −1 in a normal distribution. (Remember that the SD in a normal distribution is 1.)

28. How is the zee score used to get information from the normal distribution?

The zee score is entered into the table of values for the normal distribution and returns the corresponding area under the curve bounded by zero and the zee score. This area is identical (or nearly enough so) to the area between the sample mean and the value of interest in the sample distribution and is proportional to the percent of the sample that falls between those values. One set of tables for the normal distribution can now be used for any data sample.

29. What other information can be derived with zee scores?

You can do the calculation backward. For example, if you wanted to know the range about the mean that contains 95% of your data, you do the calculation first for a normal distribution using standard deviation units. It turns out that 95% of the values in a normal distribution fall in a range between about ±2 standard deviations from zero—roughly 47.5% above and 47.5% below. Consequently, 95% of your sample data will fall between ±2 sample standard deviations from the sample mean, provided the sample data is fairly normal. This will become important later when statistical testing is introduced.

30. How can the normal distribution relate sample and population distributions to each other?

The tie among sample distributions, population distributions, and the normal distribution is the central limit theorem. This theorem addresses the question of what happens when you draw a sample of data from a population and how well the sample reflects the distribution of data across the whole population (which you generally cannot measure and which, in turn, is the reason we are taking samples). It also addresses what happens when you draw multiple samples from the same population, how they will differ from one another, and how they will differ from the true population distribution.

31. Why is the difference among repeated samples important?

In the motorcycle example, a single sample distribution may be similar to the true population distribution. However, there is also the possibility that, by chance, you just happened to sample a lot of owners who had spent more than average that year. To be sure, you decided to repeat the sample 19 more times, for a total of 20 samples. Now not only will each of these sample distributions differ slightly from the true population distribution, but they will also differ from each other to some degree.

32. That's all very interesting but you still haven't answered the question.

True enough, but we are almost there. You could now report the mean and standard deviation of dollars spent on motorcycles that year from each group. Take all 20 mean values, plot them as a distribution, and calculate a mean value of these means. The value that these means cluster around should be very close to the true value for the population, especially as the number of samples increases. The central limit theorem says that the distribution of these means (i.e., the plot we just made) will, given enough samples, be normally distributed. Less intuitively, it says that these means will be normally distributed *even if the true population distribution was not normal to begin with.*

33. Neat trick. But what can you *do* with it?

This normal distribution of sample means will cluster around the mean of means and will have a standard deviation about that value. In this case, however, the central value they tend to cluster around is the *true population mean*—pretty useful if the whole point of sampling is that you cannot measure the whole population. The measure of dispersion of these sample means about the true population mean (analogous to the sample standard deviation about the sample mean) is estimated by the standard error of the mean and is given by the formula $SE_M = \dfrac{s}{\sqrt{n}}$, where s is the standard deviation of the sample mean and n is the sample size. Because these means are normally distributed, we can now use zee scores and the normal distribution table to infer properties of our population distribution in the same way we inferred properties of our sample distribution.

KEY POINTS: FREQUENCY DISTRIBUTIONS

1. Frequency distributions break data into categories and show how frequently each occurred.

2. They are characterized by measures of central tendency, dispersion, skew, and kurtosis.

3. They can be related to specific proportions of the sample data and to the normal distribution by the area under the curve that is defined between limiting values.

4. They tend to be normally distributed when describing the means of repeated samples, even if the original distribution was not (i.e., the central limit theorem).

5. They can be related to properties of the normal distribution through the calculation of zee scores, which are in standard deviation units.

34. What happens to the SE_M as n gets bigger?

As n gets bigger and approaches the size of the whole population, SE_M will approach zero. This makes sense because the closer your sample comes to counting everyone or everything, the less error there will be in the estimate.

35. What is the difference between a population parameter and a population statistic?

The population parameter is the true population characteristic (e.g., mean or SD) that we are trying to estimate using the process described in question 33. The population statistic is the estimated value that we calculate.

36. How do you interpret inferential statistics?

Inferential statistics will be discussed in more detail in subsequent chapters. It essentially gets at the question of how much difference there is between the population statistic and the population parameter. It also quantifies how much of that difference is due to chance, how much can be attributed to an effect of interest, and whether or not an unmeasured (but influential) "other" variable is affecting the results.

37. Can this technique be used for all types of data?

It can, to the extent that the data is normally distributed. As suggested above, the process of sampling alone tends to result in normally distributed means, which can be analyzed as I have described. Parametric testing refers to inferential tests that rely on normally distributed data. Later chapters will introduce techniques where non-normal data can be mathematically transformed so as to better approximate a normal distribution, and thus be amenable to parametric tests. There are, however, data types that are inherently non-normal. Dichotomous variables such as "alive/dead" result in a two-category frequency distribution that is not normal. There are nonparametric techniques for analyzing such data, which will also be discussed later.

PROBABILITY DISTRIBUTIONS

38. What is a probability distribution and how is it different from a frequency distribution?

Recall that, for frequency distributions, x-axis categories can be named occurrences (in the case of nominal and ordinal data) or a range of values (in the case of interval and ratio data). Within each category, the actual number of times (i.e., frequency) that the category occurred is reported on the y-axis. For each of these categories, the range of possible values for the frequency is unlimited: they can be any value between zero and infinity. However, in a probability distribution, the categories each describe a specific condition that either occurs or does not. These are referred to as dichotomous events. If you sample 100 people, the trait of motorcycle ownership is an all-or-nothing proposition. They either own one or they do not. Y-axis values thus have to be handled a little differently.

39. What are the axes in a probability distribution?

In probability distributions, the x-axis lists a series of events of interest and the y-axis is the probability that the dichotomous event described will actually occur. If 30 people out of 100 sampled answer "yes" to the question of motorcycle ownership, it does not mean that the true population must consist of 30% motorcycle owners. How likely you are to get this specific answer depends on how close this answer is to the true incidence of motorcycle ownership in the population. If the population really does have a 30% ownership rate, then the probability that 30 people of 100 sampled are motorcycle owners is likely to be relatively high. Because of sampling error, other results are possible but not as likely. In a probability distribution, one outcome on the x-axis category would be "exactly 30/100 motorcycle owners" and the y-axis value would be the probability of getting this exact result after polling 100 people.

40. **That only gives you one case. How can you make a distribution out of that?**
You cannot. Probability distributions predict the likely outcome of multiple samples by considering more than just the most probable case. You have to consider the possibility that another sample would have a different result than 30 out of 100, given a true population incidence of 0.3. Ask yourself if you would expect another 100 people surveyed to answer yes to the ownership question exactly 30 times. Your answer would be "probably not, but it should be close," and you would be correct.

41. **How does the difference from the true population value affect the probability of occurrence?**
Not surprisingly, the farther a sample is from the true population value, the less probable it is to get that answer (i.e., 34 out of 100 on the next try would not surprise you, but 80 out of 100 would). The key point is that it is not *impossible* to find, by chance, 80 motorcycle owners among 100 randomly surveyed in a population for which the base probability is 0.3. It is, however, *improbable*. The question then becomes whether you can predict the improbability of events that are that are further and further from the base incidence.

42. **How can you compute the probability of one of these unlikely cases?**
It depends on the type of data you are using. The binomial expansion is a mathematic formula that allows you to compute the probabilities for discrete, mutually exclusive, dichotomous probabilities such as the motorcycle case described above. If the outcome of interest is rare, the Poisson distribution (also a mathematical calculation) can be used. It is a good approximation of the binomial distribution and is a simpler calculation. If you are interested in the probability of outcomes that are continuous, the normal distribution can be used.

43. **Give an example of a continuous probability distribution.**
Blood pressure is a continuous variable that can, theoretically, take any value from zero to infinity. Because it is part of a biologic system that is dynamically regulated, extremely high and low values are improbable and there are normal ranges within which blood pressure is more likely to be found. It is also measured on a continuous scale with infinite divisions between integers, so the probability of any *exact* value for blood pressure is zero. The distribution of probability for *ranges* of blood pressure (and for many other biologic parameters) can be approximated by the Gaussian distribution. The mean blood pressure will be at the center of the distribution, and the probability for pressures occurring between any two values will be proportional to the area under the curve limited by those values.

44. **What variables are needed to calculate a binomial expansion?**
The binomial expansion allows you to compute the probabilities described in Question 41 using the following relevant variables: (1) the number (n) of "tries" (i.e., the number of times you test the presence or absence of the dichotomous event), (2) the number of those tries (r) that result in the event for which you want to compute the probability, and (3) the base probability (p) of the event of interest. In our example, we want to "try" 100 people and we are interested in the case in which 80 of the tries result in a "yes" answer to the ownership question.

45. **From where does the base probability come?**
Figuring the base probability is a little trickier. If our event were a coin toss and the event of interest were the coin coming up "heads," the base probability would be 0.5, no matter what actually happens when you toss. In our example, the base probability is the true percent of motorcycle owners in the entire population; to keep to our previous example, we will say 0.3 for this population and assume they are randomly distributed among the non-riders).

KEY POINTS: PROBABILITY DISTRIBUTIONS ✓

1. Probability distributions describe the likelihood of dichotomous events or traits.

2. They demonstrate how the occurrence of a dichotomous event becomes increasingly improbable (but not impossible) the further it is from the true incidence of that event or trait in the population.

3. They have a mean probability of occurrence and a standard deviation about that mean.

4. They are different for every combination of sample size and population incidence.

46. What is the calculation for the binomial expansion?
In a random sample of 100 people, there is the possibility that, by pure chance, we might just happen to include 80 motorcycle owners. This probability is given by the binomial expansion and is calculated as $\dfrac{n!}{r!\,(n-r)!}\, p^r q^{n-r}$. For our current example, n would be 100, r would be 80, and p is 0.3. (q is just $1-p$.) (Note that n! is read as "n-factorial" and is the product of all the whole numbers from 1 to n. For example, 4! would be calculated as $1 \times 2 \times 3 \times 4 = 24$.) We could repeat this calculation several times for other values of r and plot those cases on the x-axis with their corresponding probabilities on the y-axis. This would give us the binomial distribution for $n = 100$ and $p = .3$.

Figure 11-6 shows part of the results for this expansion. The overall probability for any exact result is low. However, note that the case where 30/100 people are motorcycle owners is still the highest relative probability. Answers close to 30 dominate, and the probability rapidly drops off to near zero as you move away from 30.

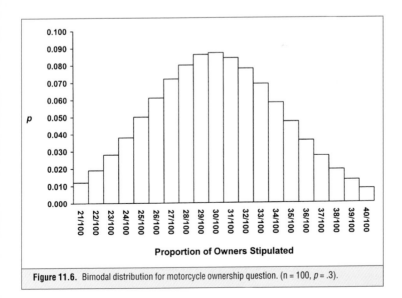

Figure 11.6. Bimodal distribution for motorcycle ownership question. ($n = 100$, $p = .3$).

47. What information can be obtained from the probability distribution thus created?

The binomial distribution shows us how improbable a dichotomous event is apt to be, the more it differs from the most probable outcome. The most probable outcome itself is analogous to the mean of a frequency distribution. The dispersion of probabilities about this mean is similarly analogous to the standard deviation and can be similarly calculated. The formula for the mean in a probability distribution is np and the standard deviation is $\sqrt{npq}$. With the standard deviation calculated, information from binomial distributions can be inferred using the normal distribution by calculating zee scores, in much the same way as we did with frequency distributions.

WEBSITES

1. http://www.sjsu.edu/faculty/gerstman/StatPrimer

2. http://www.mste.uiuc.edu/hill/dstat/dstat.html

3. http://www.davidmlane.com/hyperstat/index.html

4. http://www.emedicine.com/emerg/topic758.htm

BIBLIOGRAPHY

1. Daly LE, Bourke GJ: Interpretation and Uses of Medical Statistics, 5th ed. Oxford, Blackwell Science Ltd., 2000.
2. Kirkwood BR: Essentials of Medical Statistics. Oxford, Blackwell Science Ltd., 1988.
3. Norman GR, Streiner DL: Biostatistics: The Bare Essentials. Toronto, B.C. Decker, 2000.

CHAPTER 12

PRESENTATION OF DATA

Mark Nordness, MD

1. What is the first step in the presentation of information?

First, you must organize the information to obtain an understanding of the types and ranges of the data or results that you wish to present. Typically, a frequency distribution is constructed to help determine the best way to present the information of interest. Table 12-1 illustrates a frequency distribution of the causes of death for different age ranges in the United States in 1989. Note that, though a significant amount of information is presented, it is often difficult to visualize the shape of the distributions from a particular frame of reference. There are, however, ways to present information from tables in such a manner that the reader can readily appreciate the distribution.

TABLE 12-1.	DEATHS BY AGE AND SELECTED CAUSES OF DEATH, UNITED STATES, 1989						
Age Group (years)	Heart Disease	P&I	MVI	Diabetes	HIV	All Other	Total
<1	776	636	216	6	120	37,901	39,655
1–4	281	228	1005	15	112	5651	7292
5–14	295	122	2266	32	64	6135	8914
15–24	938	271	12,941	136	613	21,589	36,488
25–34	3462	881	10,269	687	7759	37,466	60,524
35–44	11,782	1415	6302	1432	8563	51,425	80,919
45–54	30,922	1707	3879	2784	3285	75,689	118,266
55–64	81,351	3880	3408	6942	1144	163,333	260,058
65–74	165,787	10,418	3465	13,168	327	288,059	481,224
75–84	234,318	24,022	2909	14,160	70	323,727	599,206
≥85	203,863	32,955	877	7470	12	212,181	457,358
Not stated	92	15	38	1	13	403	562
All ages	**733,867**	**76,550**	**47,575**	**46,833**	**22,082**	**1,223,559**	**2,150,466**

From Centers for Disease Control and Prevention: Principles of Epidemiology, 2nd ed. Atlanta, U.S. Department of Health and Human Services, Centers for Disease Control and Prevention, Epidemiology Program Office, Public Health Practice Program Office, 1992.

2. What is a histogram?

A histogram is a graphic representation of a given frequency distribution. In a histogram, rectangles are drawn with their bases representing a given interval, and the area of the rectangle is proportional to the number of frequency values within the interval spanned. In a true histogram, there are no spaces between the given intervals. There may well be spaces between bars on the histogram, however, if there are no values for those intervals. In practice, researchers often present histograms with small spaces between the bars to make the information clearer and more pleasing to the eye of the reader, as seen in Figure 12-1. Also note that, in Figure 12-1, the bars of the histogram may indicate different categories within the interval of interest—in this case, exposure category for the total cases of human immunodeficiency virus (HIV) infection.

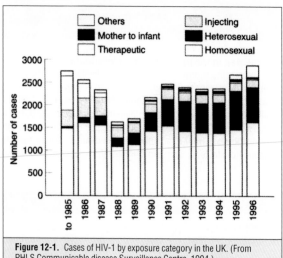

Figure 12-1. Cases of HIV-1 by exposure category in the UK. (From PHLS Communicable disease Surveillance Centre, 1994.)

3. **How large should the interval on a histogram be?**
There is no set standard. The size depends largely on the type and distribution of the data. Class intervals, however, should be of equal value. The class intervals at either end of the x-axis are often, for convenience, open-ended, or of greater total interval range. This is seen in Figure 12-1, where the first bar represents the number of cases of HIV type 1, up to 1985.

4. **How can you handle data at the extremes when constructing a histogram?**
As mentioned previously, Figure 12-1 illustrates an appropriate way to handle a few values at the extremes of the distribution. It is also acceptable to use "less than" or "greater than" a specific value at the extremes when there are a few values in these intervals.

5. **What is a weakness of histograms?**
In histograms, information about the extremes of the distributions is often lost by the use of the open-ended "less than" or "greater than" intervals at the extremes.

6. **What is a frequency polygon?**
A frequency polygon is a graph formed by joining the midpoints of the tops of histogram columns with straight lines. A frequency polygon smoothes out abrupt changes that can occur in histogram plots and helps demonstrate continuity of a variable being analyzed. Figure 12-2 demonstrates the correct method for creating a frequency polygon.

7. **Give a particularly good use of frequency polygons.**
Frequency polygons are very useful for portraying two or more distribution frequencies simultaneously. Figure 12-3 portrays three frequency polygons comparing the distribution of rabies cases.

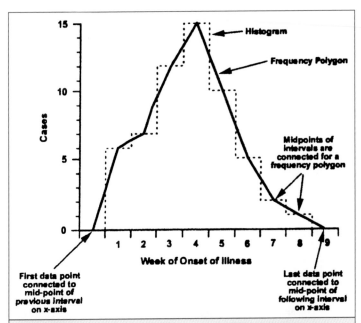

Figure 12-2. Number of reported cases of influenza-like illness by week of onset. (From Centers for Disease Control and Prevention: Principles of Epidemiology, 2nd ed. Atlanta, U.S. Department of Health and Human Services, Centers for Disease Control and Prevention, Epidemiology Program Office, Public Health Practice Program Office, 1992.)

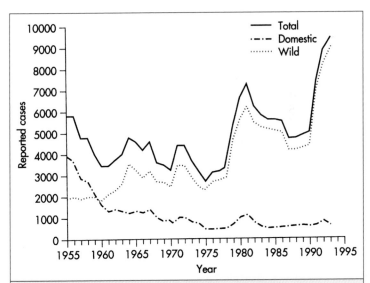

Figure 12-3. Secular trends of rabies in wild and domestic animals in the United States and Puerto Rico, 1955–1993. (From Centers for Disease and Prevention: Summary of notifiable diseases—United States, 1993. MMWR 42[53]:46, 1994.)

8. **What is a bar diagram?**

A bar diagram (i.e., bar chart) is a graphic representation of discrete data. Different categories or classifications are represented on one axis, and the frequency count is represented on the other. Because the categories are discrete and mutually exclusive, the bar chart should always be represented with a space between bars. Like a histogram, the area of the bar is proportional to the count. Figure 12-4 is an example of a bar chart.

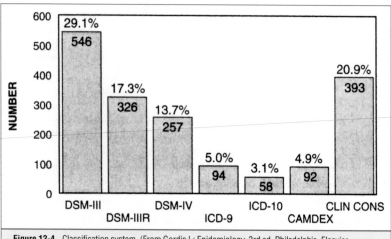

Figure 12-4. Classification system. (From Gordis L: Epidemiology, 3rd ed. Philadelphia, Elsevier-Saunders, 2004.)

9. **What is a geographic distribution map?**

Also known as an epidemiologic map, a case map, or a choroplethic map, this type of presentation displays quantitative information in defined geographic areas. Areas may be represented in any convenient and meaningful way; often counties, states, or countries are used (Fig. 12-5).

10. **What is a stem-and-leaf diagram?**

The stem-and-leaf diagram, invented by John Tukey, is a unique method of summarizing data without losing the individual data points. The stems in these diagrams are the left-hand digits of the numeric data, and the leaves are the last digit to the right of the stem. The frequency of each stem value (which is the number of leaves) is given in a separate column. Table 12-2 shows an example of a stem-and-leaf diagram in the upper left area. Here, the stem digits represent 10s; thus, 3 is equal to 30, 4 is equal to 40, and so on. The leaves are the 1s of the column digits. Therefore, looking at the 7 from the stem column, the leaves of 0 and 7 represent values of 70 and 77, respectively.

11. **How is a stem-and-leaf diagram like a histogram?**

A stem-and-leaf diagram is essentially a histogram on its side, with stem values representing the intervals and leaves representing the frequency count in the interval. Note that it is important to represent repeated values each time that they appear in the frequency distribution. For example, in Table 12-2, the two zeroes in the 6-stem represent a value of 60 occurring twice.

12. **What is a box-and-whisker plot?**

A box-and-whisker plot is a visual representation of data with a box made at the value of the median, represented by a middle line, with two divisions. The vertical height of the lower division represents the first quartile (i.e., 25th percentile), and the upper division represents the third

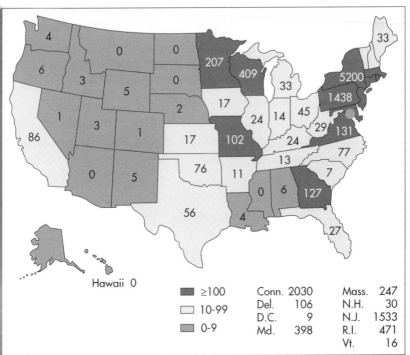

Figure 12-5. Geographic distribution of Lyme disease cases in the United States, 1994. (From Centers for Disease Control and Prevention: Lyme disease—United States, 1994. MMWR 44[24]:459–461, 1995.)

quartile (i.e., 75th percentile). The width of the box is arbitrary. Vertical lines are drawn from the minimum value to the lower box and from the maximum value to the upper box. A box-and-whisker plot is represented to the right of the stem-and-leaf diagram in Table 12-2.

13. **What is an *outside value* in a box-and-whisker plot?**
An outside value is defined as either a value that is smaller than the lower quartile minus 1.5 times the interquartile range, or a value larger than the upper quartile plus 1.5 times the interquartile range.

14. **What is a *far-out value* in a box and whisker plot?**
A far-out value is defined as a value that is either smaller than the lower quartile minus 3 times the interquartile range, or larger than the upper quartile plus 3 times the interquartile range.

15. **What is an advantage of a box-and-whisker plot?**
A box-and-whisker plot offers the ability to display all of the data with a statistic summary.

16. **What is a pie diagram?**
A pie diagram (Fig. 12-6) is a visually effective and simple method of representing data. It is a circular diagram divided into segments, each of which represents the frequency of a category. The total of the slices of the pie must add up to 100%. Often the segments are ordered by size, from largest to smallest, in a clockwise direction. A general rule of thumb is not to have more than five or six slices in a chart to prevent it from becoming too cluttered. Small slices may also

TABLE 12-2.   STEM–AND–LEAF DIAGRAM AND BOXPLOT

Stem Leaf	#	Boxplot
9 0	1	0
8 1	1		
7 07	2		
6 0023479	7	+-----+
5 234788	6	*--+--*
4 14677889	8	+-----+
3 1	1		

   ----+ ----+----+----+

Multiply Stem.Leaf by 10**+ 1

	Quantiles (Percentiles)		
100% Max	90	99%	90
75% Q3	64	95%	81
50% Med	57.5	90%	77
25% Q1	48	10%	44
0% Min	31	5%	41
		1%	31
Range	59		
Q3-Q1	16		
Mode	47		

From Jekel JF, Katz DL, Elmore JG: Epidemiology, Biostatistics, and Preventive Medicine, 2nd ed. Philadelphia, W.B. Saunders, 2001.

be pulled out and represented in a sort of sub-pie arrangement to show greater detail, as demonstrated in Figure 12-6.

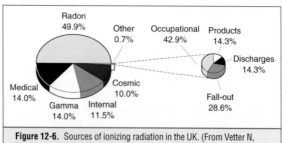

Figure 12-6. Sources of ionizing radiation in the UK. (From Vetter N, Matthews I: Epidemiology and Public Health Medicine. Philadelphia, Churchill Livingstone, 1999.)

17. **What is a disadvantage of pie charts?**
It can be very difficult to see the difference in slice sizes when data values are similar. For ease in interpretation, the pie slices should be labeled with the actual values.

KEY POINTS: PRESENTATION OF DATA

1. Histograms are an effective way to illustrate frequency counts of continuous data divided into intervals.

2. Information regarding extreme data points is often lost in histograms.

3. Frequency polygons are constructed by connecting the dots from the midpoints of the individual histogram bars.

4. Bar charts are useful for presenting counts of discrete data.

5. Stem-and-leaf charts summarize data without losing individual data points.

6. Pie charts are useful for showing the relative distributions that together represent 100% of the outcome of interest.

18. **What is a line graph?**

A line graph is a useful method of displaying data over a period of time. Often an occurrence rate of some type is represented on the y-axis over a given period of time on the x-axis. An important issue in the use of a line graph is showing a broad-enough interval on the x-axis to prevent an incorrect conclusion from being drawn with respect to trends over time. Figure 12-7 and Figure 12-8 show a line graph representing death rates among men and women from ages 25–44 in the United States from 1982–2000.

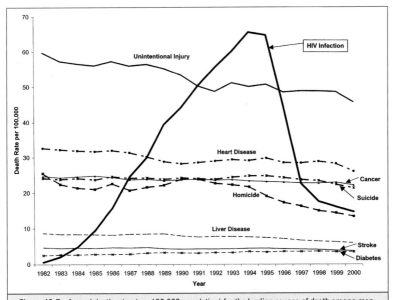

Figure 12-7. Annual death rates (per 100,000 population) for the leading causes of death among men ages 25–44. (From Gordis L: Epidemiology, 3rd ed. Philadelphia, Elsevier-Saunders, 2004. Drawn from data prepared by Richard M. Selik, MD, Division of HIV/AIDS Prevention, Centers for Disease Control and Prevention, 2003.)

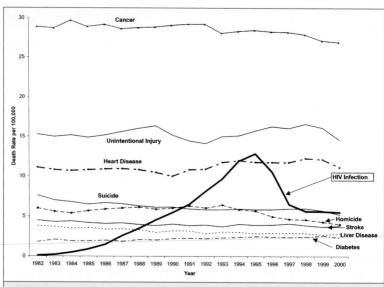

Figure 12-8. Annual death rates (per 100,000 population) for leading causes of death among women ages 25–44. (From Gordis L: Epidemiology, 3rd ed. Philadelphia, Elsevier-Saunders, 2004. Drawn from data prepared by Richard M. Selik, MD, Division of HIV/AIDS Prevention, Centers for Disease Control and Prevention, 2003.)

19. **Can cartoons and images be used to represent differences in data?**
    This technique is used more often by marketers than by scientists and is fraught with concerns of misrepresentation. As a simple example, examine the two cubes in Figure 12-9. The length of one side of the larger cube is approximately twice the length of the smaller. Would this be a fair representation of a tomato seed that yields twice as much produce as its competitor? Of course not—we know that, in fact, the area of one face of the bigger cube is four times greater than the smaller and that the volume is eight times larger. Be suspicious of data or claims represented in a pictorial fashion.

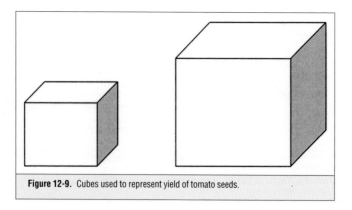

Figure 12-9. Cubes used to represent yield of tomato seeds.

WEBSITES

1. http://www.acepidemiology.org
2. http://www.apha.org/public_health/epidemiology.htm

BIBLIOGRAPHY

1. Centers for Disease Control: Principles of Epidemiology, 2nd ed. Atlanta, U.S. Department of Health and Human Services, Centers for Disease Control and Prevention, Epidemiology Program Office, Public Health Practice Program Office,1992.
2. Daly LE, Bourke GJ: Interpretation and Uses of Medical Statistics, 5th ed. Oxford, Blackwell Science Ltd., 2000.
3. Gordis L: Epidemiology, 3rd ed. Philadelphia, W.B. Saunders, 2004.
4. Jekel JF, Katz DL, Elmore JG: Epidemiology, Biostatistics, and Preventive Medicine. Philadelphia, W.B. Saunders, 2001, pp 20–39.
5. Kirkwood BR: Essentials of Medical Statistics. Oxford, Blackwell Science Ltd., 1988.
6. Last JM (ed): A Dictionary of Epidemiology, 4th ed. Oxford, Oxford University Press, 2001.
7. Rothman KJ, Greenland S (eds): Modern Epidemiology. Philadelphia, Lippincott Williams & Wilkins, 1998, pp 435–447.
8. Torrence ME: Understanding Epidemiology. St Louis, Mosby, 1997.
9. Vetter N, Matthews I: Epidemiology and Public Health Medicine. Philadelphia, Churchill Livingstone, 1999.

CHAPTER 13

HYPOTHESIS TESTING

Neal Andrew Naito, MD, MPH

1. **What is hypothesis testing?**

   Hypothesis testing is a statistical method usually used when a comparison has to be made, such as between two drugs or two procedures. It is a process whereby the statistical importance of an investigation finding is determined by calculating the value of the chosen test statistic, which is taken from a population sample, and seeing if the value is equal to or greater than the preset significance level. If it is, the result is termed *statistically significant.*

2. **How do researchers and clinicians use the results of hypothesis testing?**

   With the present emphasis on evidence-based medicine, it is important for clinicians to understand hypothesis testing because it is the starting point for knowing whether research results are potentially applicable clinically. If statistical significance is achieved, then deciding whether a finding is clinically significant can be considered. A shortcoming of clinical research studies is that conclusions often do not consider clinical significance fully and, instead, heavily base the importance of the findings on mainly statistical results.

3. **When is a result "statistically significant?"**

   As previously mentioned, a result is statistically significant when the test statistic (e.g., t, z, or χ^2) is greater than or equal to the significance level. The test statistic is chosen based on the type of data being evaluated. By contrast, the significance level is predetermined by the researcher and is not dependent on the data. By convention, the significance level is termed α and is usually set at 0.05, although 0.1 and 0.01 are sometimes used as well. At 0.05, there is a 1 in 20 chance that the null hypothesis may be rejected when, in fact, it is true (i.e., type I error).

   Although similar to α, the *p*-value differs subtly by representing the probability that the test statistic will be equally or more extreme than the one actually calculated, given that the null hypothesis is true. The *p*-value will differ from one sample to the next.

4. **What is the null hypothesis?**

   The null hypothesis (H_0) represents the actual hypothesis to be tested. It is a somewhat artificial framework through which to properly define the research question in order to use the appropriate statistic analysis. The basic premise of the null hypothesis is that the study result will show no change or difference. In clinical research, a typical null hypothesis states that there is no difference in treatment results between a new drug and a placebo. The null hypothesis is often misinterpreted since hypothesizing no difference or change is counterintuitive to the actual objective of the research.

5. **Define the alternate hypothesis.**

   The alternate hypothesis (H_A) is the opposite supposition of the null hypothesis. It is the actual research question of interest, stated in a particular form that can be tested indirectly. In the above example, the alternate hypothesis would state that there is a difference in treatment outcomes between the new drug and a placebo.

6. **What does it mean if the null hypothesis is rejected or accepted?**

   The goal of most research is to reject the null hypothesis so that the alternate hypothesis can then be accepted. Acceptance of the null hypothesis, by definition, leads to rejection of the alternate hypothesis. In more essential terms, if the null hypothesis is rejected, then a statistically meaningful difference was found in the study.

Acceptance or rejection is based on whether the test statistic is equal to or greater than the significance level, which was chosen before the study began and, by convention, is usually 0.05. The significance level is the probability of rejecting a true null hypothesis, or, in plain English, finding a statistical difference where, in fact, none exists.

7. **How does one-tailed testing differ from two-tailed testing?**
These terms refer to whether the effect that is being studied can occur in only one direction (e.g., an increase, a decrease, an improvement, or a harm) or in any direction. An example of a two-tailed test is the investigation of a new drug, which may be helpful or harmful. In comparison, studying the effects of smoking on longevity would be a one-tailed test since there is no evidence that smoking improves health over the long run.

8. **What are the advantages and disadvantages of using a one-tailed test?**
The major advantage of a one-tailed test is that, generally, a smaller number of study subjects are needed to reach a certain power, as compared to a two-tailed test. Also, the difference noted between a baseline and a hypothesized value, to reach the necessary significance level is smaller with a one-tailed than with a two-tailed test.

A disadvantage of the one-tail test is the loss of the ability to test for unanticipated results.

9. **How does a researcher decide between a one-tailed and a two-tailed test?**
Deciding on a one-tailed (Fig. 13-1) or a two-tailed (Fig. 13-2) testing strategy must be done at the beginning of developing a study design, and the decision should not be switched once data collection is underway. A two-tailed test is most often used because researchers frequently need the flexibility to test for unanticipated effects in the opposite direction of what was expected.

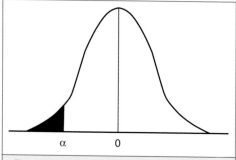

Figure 13-1. Graphic representation of a one-tailed test.

10. **What are the steps in hypothesis testing?**
1. Develop null and alternative hypotheses from the research question being investigated.
2. Determine an appropriate test statistic (e.g., t, z, F, or χ^2) to be used, based on the research sample groups chosen.
3. Choose the appropriate significance level (i.e., $\alpha = 0.05$) for performing the statistic test, and determine the test statistic value to achieve it.
4. Perform the calculation to determine the value of the test statistic.
5. Draw and state the conclusion: whether to accept or reject the null hypothesis.

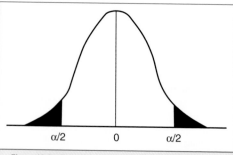

Figure 13-2. Graphic representation of a two-tailed test.

11. **Define type I error and α.**

A type I error is committed by not accepting the null hypothesis when, in fact, it is true. The probability (p) of making a type I error is designated by the symbol α. The significance level is the value for which α is set at in hypothesis testing (usually 0.05). It is an arbitrary value chosen as the cut-off point for which the *p*-value is considered significant or not significant.

$$\alpha = p \text{ (type I error)}$$

Another way to phrase the description of a type I error is that the finding is due to chance.

12. **Give an example of a type I error.**

A clinic researcher reaches the conclusion that a medication lowers blood pressure more than a placebo by an amount that is statistically significant when, in fact, the medication is not more effective than the placebo.

13. **What is a type II error and β?**

Accepting the null hypothesis when, in fact, it is false is a type II error. The symbol β denotes the probability of making a type II error.

$$\beta = p \text{(type II error)}$$

KEY POINTS: BASIC DEFINITIONS

1. Null hypothesis: the premise that the study result will show no change or difference.

2. Alternate hypothesis: the opposite supposition of the null hypothesis (i.e., the study result will show change or difference).

3. One-tailed testing: the effect of the study can occur in only one direction (e.g., increase, decrease, an improvement, or a harm).

4. Two-tailed testing: the effect of the study can occur in any direction (e.g., the effect may be helpful or harmful).

5. Alpha (α): the probability of making a type I error (i.e., rejecting the null hypothesis when, in fact, it is true).

6. Beta (β): the probability of making a type II error (i.e., accepting the null hypothesis when, in fact, it is false).

14. **What is the term for the equation 1−β?**

Power is the special term given to the probability of not accepting a false null hypothesis, which is equal to 1−β.

15. **Give an example of a type II error.**

A cardiology researcher conducts an animal experiment to determine whether cardiac muscle is affected by a new drug and finds the effect does not differ from placebo. However, upon conducting a further study with more animal subjects, the cardiology researcher finds that the drug does differ from placebo in its effect on cardiac muscle.

16. **What is the relationship between α and β?**

In order to make α and β as small as possible, α is usually fixed first.

Because β is inversely related to α, β will tend to get larger if α is made smaller at a fixed sample size. Consequently, for any designated α, increased sample sizes will lead to statistic tests with greater powers and smaller β values. (See Table 13-1.)

TABLE 13–1. RELATIONSHIP BETWEEN α AND β

Test of Significance Conclusion	Population Reality	
	H_0 True	H_0 Not True (H_A True)
Accept H_0	Correct decision	Decision not correct, type II error (probability = β)
Do not accept H_0	Incorrect decision, type I error (probability = α)	Correct decision (probability = $1-\beta$ = power)

17. **What is the p-value?**

    The p-value is the probability of obtaining a result equal to or more extreme than what was actually observed, assuming the null hypothesis. It measures the strength of evidence against the null hypothesis. The smaller the p-value, the stronger the evidence against H_0, which means rejecting H_0 is not likely due to chance alone if the p-value is less than or equal to α. (See Fig. 13-3.)

    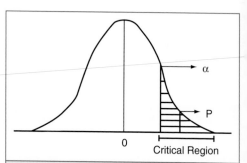

    Figure 13-3. Graphic representation of the relationship between α and the p-value. The area under the bell-shaped curve represents the probability of all outcomes stemming from the null hypothesis. The critical region is the tail area encompassing those values of the test statistic (e.g., z, t, χ^2, etc.) that equal a p-value $\leq \alpha$.

18. **Describe some of the pitfalls associated with use of the p-value.**

    One of the criticisms of the p-value is that it does not convey information in regard to the size of the observed effect. A small effect in a study with a large sample size can have the same p-value as a large effect in a small study. Another problem is that the more variables or endpoints in a study, the more likely one of them will come up statistically significant by chance alone, making the test's clinical significance circumspect. (Remember: a p-value of .05 means that, by chance alone, every 1 out of 20 times an event or finding will occur.) Similarly, subgroup analysis, as well as repeated analysis of data during accrual with cessation of the experiment or trial when statistic significance is reached, is likely to lead to incorrect conclusions.

19. **What is data mining?**

    Data mining refers to the potentially inappropriate use of repeated subgroup analysis on a data set until a relationship that is statistically significant is found. Remember that, by convention, at $\alpha = 0.05$, there is a 1 in 20 chance that a finding will be statistically significant when, in fact, it is not (i.e., a type I error). Consequently, if one does repeated subgroup analysis of a data set, any findings of statistical significance should be confirmed, if possible, by a dedicated research study of their own.

20. **How should p-values be reported?**

    Another important aspect of the p-value is in its reporting in clinic studies. Reporting of the actual p-value is becoming more prevalent because it gives the reviewer of the study more sense of the degree of statistical significance. For instance, if a p-value is found to be .06, it is more informative for that result to be reported, rather than simply stating that statistical significance was not achieved.

If the study hypothesis was biologically plausible, one might want to investigate the hypothesis further before deciding whether it is true. Conversely, one has to be careful of overstating the importance of a finding by saying the result was "approaching statistical significance" with the same $p = .06$.

KEY POINTS: THE p-VALUE

1. Defined as the probability of obtaining a result equal to or more extreme than what was actually observed, assuming the null hypothesis.

2. The α value is fixed, whereas the p-value is calculated and will vary.

3. Measures the strength of evidence against the null hypothesis.

4. The smaller the p-value, the stronger the evidence against the null hypothesis (e.g., a p-value of .05 means that in 1 of 20 times an event or finding will occur by chance alone).

5. Major disadvantage: the p-value does not convey information about the size of the observed effect (i.e., a small effect in a large sample can have the same p-value as a large effect in a small sample).

6. Other disadvantage: the more variables or endpoints tested for in a study, the more likely that one of them will be statistically significant by chance alone.

21. **Explain power.**
Power is the probability of not accepting the null hypothesis when it is false and the alternative hypothesis is true—that is, *finding a significant difference when it truly exists.* It is the complement of β and is equal to $1-\beta$. It differs from α and β in that it does not address the probability of committing a specific error, but instead the probability of reaching the right conclusion with a statistical test.

22. **Why is power important?**
Its importance relates to estimating, as accurately as possible, the sample size needed for a study to achieve statistical significance, if it exists. Power helps to avoid the problem of inconclusive or negative results when, actually, one would find statistical significance if the sample size were larger. Moreover, an accurate estimation of the number of study subjects needed to carry out a research investigation is important in order to budget appropriately the financial resources needed to complete the investigation.

23. **What is a standard value for power?**
By convention, the power is set at 0.80 for sample size analyses. Higher values of power are desirable whenever financially and logistically feasible. As mentioned previously, other factors that need to be considered when setting sample size include the value of α (usually at 0.05), the potential directions of the effects of the test (i.e., one-tailed vs. two-tailed), and the magnitude of response rates to be detected.

$$\text{Power} = P(\text{not accept } H_0 \mid H_0 \text{ false}) = P(\text{find } H_A \text{ true} \mid H_A \text{ true})$$
$$= P(\text{not accept } H_0 \mid H_A \text{ true})$$

24. **Which variables affect power?**
Power is affected by the same properties that affect the computation to accept or reject H_0 and H_A (i.e., the calculation of the chosen test statistic); the variables affected depend on which type of data is being compared. The general formula for calculating a test statistic is the following:

$$\text{test statistic} = \frac{\text{sample estimate} - \text{hypothesized value}}{\text{standard error of the sample estimate}}$$

Using the z statistic, the general formula would be as follows:

$$z = \frac{x - \mu}{\sigma / \sqrt{n}}$$

where x = the sample estimate, μ = the hypothesized value, and $\sigma / \sqrt{n}$ = the standard error of x. From these formulas, it is easy to see how the power would be affected by the effect size being tested ($x - \mu$), the sample size (n), and the variability (standard deviation) among the samples (σ).

25. **Give an example of a power calculation.**

You are a researcher studying the effects of a medication on raising high-density lipoprotein (HDL) cholesterol levels in women. You would like to perform a power calculation of your proposed study. Your research budget allows you to recruit 100 study participants. You hypothesize that men taking the medication will have a higher HDL by 10 points than those who do not. Previous research results show that men in your study population have, in general, an HDL of 36. For the purpose of this example, you have determined $\sigma = 30$. You decide an α of 0.05 is acceptable, which corresponds to a z of 1.65.

$$1.65 = \frac{x - 36}{30 / \sqrt{100}} \qquad x = 40.95$$

$$z = \frac{40.95 - 46}{30 / \sqrt{100}} = -1.653$$

$$\beta = 0.0465$$

$$\text{power} = 1 - \beta = 1 - .047 = 0.953$$

Thus, the chance is 95% that a 10-point difference in the HDL exists among women taking the medication will be detected by the statistical test.

26. **What is the difference between "statistically significant" and "clinically significant?" Why is it important?**

A good clinic research study should make clear the sequential but separate relationship between statistical and clinical significance. A finding of statistical significance should not automatically lead to the conclusion of clinical importance. Hypothesis testing only indirectly assesses the underlying truth of a finding by limiting the number of times a wrong conclusion is reached. Biologic plausibility, effect size, patient population applicability, and cost are some of the factors that one has to consider in determining whether a statistically significant finding (i.e., positive result) is also relevant from a clinical standpoint. For example, in drug trials involving cancer therapies, prolongation of life for several months on the experimental medication versus placebo is frequently found to be statistically significant. Yet, the previously mentioned factors need to be considered before concluding whether the new therapy is clinically significant.

27. **What are the implications of study findings that are "statistically not significant?" Does it mean the negative results are also "clinically not significant?"**

The opposite also holds true when a difference between two study populations is found to be not statistically significant, even though it is biologically plausible. In this case, as in many other studies reported in the medical literature, the study probably had inadequate power, resulting from a low sample size. Failure to perform an adequate power analysis is considered by some to be unethical since research subjects are needlessly exposed to interventions. If the study hypothesis is biologically plausible, one may want to investigate the hypothesis further before deciding whether it is true. Conversely, one has to be careful of overstating the importance of a finding by saying that the result was "approaching statistical significance" with the same $p = .06$.

28. **What is a meta-analysis? How is it useful?**

Meta-analysis is the research technique whereby different, smaller studies can be screened for compatibility and then combined using standardized criteria to create a larger sample size, which translates into increased power. This increased power allows a more accurate estimation of the statistical significance of an intervention's effect. Nonetheless, a meta-analysis is not a substitute for large, randomized, controlled clinic trials. There are numerous examples in the medical literature in which findings differed between the two types of studies investigating the same problem.

29. **When are underpowered studies justifiable?**

Underpowered studies can probably be justified in two settings: (1) investigating a rare disease, and (2) performing pilot studies on new drugs or therapies. By their very nature, the patient populations of rare diseases are small, and accruing enough subjects to run a clinic trial to achieve statistical significance based on preliminary power calculations may not be possible. Consequently, in conducting such a study, the reporting becomes important. The use of confidence intervals is preferable to p-values because they allow interpretation of the possible effect size, even if statistical significance is not achieved. (This will be further explained later in this chapter.) In regard to pilot studies, the issues are usually cost and safety, in that the number of research subjects is intentionally kept smaller in comparison to a regular clinic trial. This approach limits the cost of the trial, if a new drug or therapy proves ineffective, and also minimizes the harm, in terms of the number of study participants exposed, if there is a side effect.

30. **What is the standard error (SE)?**

A measurement of the spread of sample data means. It is calculated as the standard deviation (SD) of a population of sample means divided by the square root of the sample size (N).

$$SE = \frac{SD}{\sqrt{N}}$$

By contrast, the SD is a measurement of the spread of data based on individual observations. The importance of the SE lies in its use in calculating confidence intervals.

31. **Which statistic measure of variation is generally best for reporting data: standard deviation or standard error?**

In presenting data, either the mean and the standard deviation or the mean and the standard error are often used. However, the use of the standard deviation is encouraged over the use of the standard error. Using the standard error can be disadvantageous because it is based on the sample size and can be changed simply by manipulating N, and also because it is based on means and not individual observations. This latter problem is best highlighted in journal articles, in which the use of the interval mean ±2 SE for reporting of findings is often mistakenly interpreted as encompassing 95% of all individual data results involved in a study.

32. **What is a confidence interval?**

A confidence interval is a range of likely values defined by upper and lower endpoints (i.e., confidence limits) within which the true value of an unknown population parameter is likely to fall, based on a preset confidence level. The general expression for confidence interval is

Confidence interval = point estimate ± (confidence multiplier × SE)

For the 90%, 95%, and 99% confidence levels, the multiplier is 1.645, 1.96, and 2.576, respectively. The term *confidence* is used instead of probability because the true value of the population parameter either falls within the interval or does not eliminate. Thus, in practical terms, a 95% confidence interval for a given parameter—for instance, the population mean, μ—implies that 95% of similarly constructed intervals will contain μ.

33. **What are the advantages of using confidence intervals versus *p*-values?**
Many medical journals now require the use of confidence intervals because they provide more information than the *p*-value in the setting of both positive and negative results. For example, instead of reporting that the difference in control of blood pressure by drug A versus drug B is statistically significant, it is more helpful to report the confidence intervals of each drug so that one can see the effect size (i.e., the amount by which the drugs could differ). Conversely, if the findings are not statistically significant, confidence intervals can give an indication as to whether there is a potential for clinic significance if further studies are pursued, which usually happens when a larger sample size is needed. When using the same population for analysis, the inferences drawn from confidence intervals and hypothesis testing are compatible with each other.

34. **How can you affect the width (i.e., precision) of the confidence interval?**
   - Choose a smaller confidence level.
   - Reduce the standard deviation by using a different sampling technique, such as a stratified approach.
   - Take larger samples to increase N.

   Adjusting any of these factors, alone or together, can decrease the width of the confidence interval.

WEBSITES

1. http://www.apha.org/public_health/epidemiology.htm
2. http://www.amstat.org/sections/epi/SIE_Home.htm

BIBLIOGRAPHY

1. Browner WS, Newman TB, Cummings SR, et al: Getting ready to estimate sample size: Hypothesis and underlying principles. In Hulley SB, Cummings SR (eds): Designing Clinical Research: An Epidemiologic Approach. Baltimore, Williams & Wilkins, 1988, pp 128–150, 232–236.
2. Colton T: Statistics in Medicine. Boston, Little, Brown & Company, 1974, pp 99–150.
3. Daly LE: Confidence limits made easy: Interval estimation using a substitution method. Am J Epidemiol 147(8):783–790, 1998.
4. Dawson B, Trapp RG: Basic and Clinical Biostatistics, 3rd ed. New York, Lange, 2001, pp 63–135.
5. Goodman SN: Toward evidence-based medical statistics. 1: The P-value fallacy. Ann Intern Med 130:995–1004, 1999.
6. Guyatt G, Jaeschke R, Heddle N, et al: Basic statistics for clinicians: 2. Interpreting study results: Confidence intervals. Can Med Assoc J 152(2):169–173, 1995.
7. Halpern SD, Karlawish JH, Berlin JA: The continuing unethical conduct of underpowered clinical trials. JAMA 288(3):358–36, 2002.
8. Knapp RG, Miller MC: Clinical Epidemiology and Biostatistics. Baltimore, Williams & Wilkins, 1992, pp 167–208.

CHAPTER 14

PROBABILITY AND SAMPLING

Jonathan M. Lieske, MD, MPH

PROBABILITY

1. **What is probability?**
   Probability is a quantification of the likelihood, or relative frequency, of occurrence of a given event or set of events, over a sequence of unlimited random trials done under similar conditions. Probability compares the number of desirable events (A) to the total number of trials during which the event may occur (N).

2. **How is probability calculated?**
   The standard equation for a probability calculation is P(event) = A/N, where P(event) is the probability of the studied event occurring, A is the number of times the desired event actually occurs, and N is the total number of trials during which A may occur. The probability of A occurring is expressed as a percentage that is never greater than 1 (100%) or less than 0 (0%).

3. **A physician in family practice for 20 years has followed 1000 patients diagnosed with disease Y. Based on his sample (Table 14-1), what is the probability that a randomly selected patient with disease Y will be a male of any age? An elderly patient of either sex? An elderly male?**
   In Table 14-1, the probability of randomly choosing a patient with any of the selected characteristics can be determined easily by simply identifying the correct entry on the spreadsheet and dividing by the appropriate denominator. From the table we find
   - P(male) = 350/1000 = 0.35
   - P(elderly) = 600/1000 = 0.6
   - P(male, elderly) = 200/1000 = 0.2

TABLE 14-1. DEMOGRAPHIC DISTRIBUTION OF PATIENTS WITH DISEASE Y			
Age	Female	Male	Total
Young	250	150	400
Elderly	400	200	600
Total	650	350	1000

4. **Describe the difference between probability and odds.**
   Odds are also a measurement of the likelihood of occurrence of an event; however, odds are a ratio of the probability that an event occurs to the probability that the event does *not* occur:

   Odds = (probability of occurrence)/(probability of nonoccurrence)

5. **When rolling a single unbiased die, what is the probability of rolling a 1?**
   Given the fact there are six sides to the die and only one side with a 1, there are six possible outcomes (1, 2, 3, 4, 5, 6), one of which (1) is the desired event. The other five potential outcomes (2, 3, 4, 5, 6) are considered undesirable events. The *probability* of rolling a 1 = the number of desirable events divided by the total number of possible events = 1/6 = 16.67%.

6. **What are the odds of rolling a 1?**
   The *odds* of rolling a 1 are the probability of the desirable event (i.e., rolling a 1) divided by the probability of undesirable events (i.e., rolling anything besides 1). In this case,

   $$Odds = (probability\ of\ rolling\ a\ 1)/(probability\ of\ not\ rolling\ a\ 1)$$
   $$= (1/6)/(5/6)$$
   $$= 1/5$$
   $$= 0.2$$

7. **If the probability that a given event will occur is known, how are the odds calculated?**
   Probability may be easily converted into odds using the following equation:

   $$Odds = probability/(1 - probability)$$

   Consider an example of a coin toss in which you have called "heads." Assuming that you are flipping an unbiased coin, the probability of the result being heads = probability of tails = 1/2 = 0.5. In calculating the odds of tossing heads, the equation yields

   $$Odds = 0.5/(1 - 0.5) = 0.5/0.5 = 1$$

   The equation makes intuitive sense because the probability of occurrence (i.e., heads) is equal to the probability of nonoccurrence (i.e., tails), making the ratio 1. Therefore, when the odds are 1, there is an equal chance of occurrence and nonoccurrence.

8. **Conversely, if the odds that a given event will occur are known, how is probability calculated?**
   Odds may be easily converted into probability using the following equation:

   $$Probability = odds/(1 + odds)$$

   Using numbers from the previous example of rolling a 1 on a single roll of a die,

   $$Probability = 0.2/(1 + 0.2) = 0.1667$$

9. **Define joint probability.**
   Joint probability is the probability of two events occurring together. The joint probability of events A and B occurring together is annotated as P(A, B). This notation was used in question 3 when we considered the probability that a person diagnosed with disease Y is both male and elderly: P(male, elderly).

10. **What is marginal probability?**
    Marginal probability is the probability that a single event will occur, without consideration of any other event.

11. **As it relates to probability, what is meant by independent events?**
    When considering the probability of occurrence of multiple events, the probability of occurrence of one event is *not* influenced by the outcome of a prior event if the two events are independent. Two events A and B are therefore independent *if* the occurrence of A has *no effect* on the occurrence of the other event, B.

12. **What is an example of the concept of independent events?**

The coin flip is a good vehicle to explain the concept. Again, assuming an unbiased coin, the results of all previous flips mean nothing when determining the probability of flipping a "head," which is 0.5 or 50%. If 5 heads (or 500) were consecutively flipped immediately prior to the flip of interest, the probability of heads on the next flip would be unchanged.

13. **What is conditional probability?**

Conditional probability is the probability of occurrence of one event (A), *given that a second event (B) has occurred*. The conditional probability of A occurring, given B, is written $P(A \mid B)$ and is read as "the probability of A given B." The equation for determining conditional probability is as follows:

$$P(A \mid B) = \text{(number of times A and B occur jointly)/(number of times B occurs)}$$

14. **If events A and B are independent, how is the conditional probability affected?**

If the events A and B are independent, the equation in question 13 reduces to $P(A \mid B) = P(A)$. This again makes intuitive sense because the fact that B has occurred has no bearing on the occurrence of A in considering two independent events.

15. **Using the spreadsheet from Table 14-1, what is the probability that a patient diagnosed with disease Y will be female, *given* that the patient is elderly [P(female | elderly)]?**

This is an example of conditional probability. Using Table 14-1, you can easily appreciate that we are actually concerned about the subpopulation of elderly patients because the probability of being female is based on the condition that the patient is elderly.

There are a total of 400 females who are elderly out of a total of 600 elderly patients. Hence, P(female | elderly) = (the number of times that female and elderly occur jointly)/(the number of times elderly occurs):

$$P(\text{female} \mid \text{elderly}) = 400/600 = 0.67$$

16. **A player needs to draw two cards of the same suit in order to win a card game. Given that the first card he draws is a spade and is not replaced into the deck after being drawn, what is the probability that the player will draw a second spade?**

This is again an example of conditional probability. Given that the deck consists of 52 cards with 13 cards of each suit, if the player first draws a spade, there are now only 12 spades remaining in the deck. Therefore, the conditional probability of drawing a second spade, given his first draw, may be annotated as follows:

$$P(\text{drawing second spade} \mid \text{initial spade}) = 12/51 = 0.235$$

17. **What is the probability of drawing a spade from a deck of cards *after* drawing a spade from a deck of cards and then replacing the card?**

These two events are independent of each other, with the drawing of the first spade having no influence on the second draw. Therefore, the probability in question is the same as that of simply drawing a spade from a deck of cards = 13/52 = 0.25.

18. **Describe the relationship between conditional probability and relative risk.**

Consider B an outcome of interest and A a potential risk factor for outcome B.

The relative risk of B given A is defined by the following equation:

$$\text{Relative risk} = [P(B \mid A)]/[P(B \mid \bar{A})]$$

where P(B | A) is the probability of event B, given that event A occurs, and P(B | Ā) is the probability of event B, given that event A does not occur. If the two events are independent, the relative risk will be 1, which indicates that A is in fact not a risk factor for B. However, the greater the effect of A on B, the further the relative risk will be from 1.

19. **Consider a clinic example using fictitious data for a sample of patients who have had one positive Hemoccult test.**

    When serial Hemoccult testing is performed to screen for colon cancer, the probability of carcinoma (event B) if a retest Hemoccult test is positive (event A) is 0.143; alternatively, the probability of carcinoma in a patient with a negative Hemoccult retest (event A does not occur) is 0.01. Therefore, the relative risk of carcinoma for those with a second positive Hemoccult compared with those whose second Hemoccult is negative can be calculated as follows:

$$\text{Relative risk} = [P(B \mid A)]/[P(B \mid \bar{A})] = 0.143/0.01 = 14.3$$

    This result is significantly greater than 1, demonstrating the fact that dependence exists between events A and B and supporting the use of serial Hemoccult testing for colon cancer screening.

20. **What is mutual exclusivity?**

    The concept of mutual exclusivity states that two events (A and B) are mutually exclusive if they *cannot* occur simultaneously. The probability of two mutually exclusive events (A and B) occurring at the same time is 0. For instance, flipping a coin one time and having both a "head" and a "tail" at the same time is impossible; thus, the probability of this occurrence is 0. Therefore, simultaneous "heads" and "tails" are mutually exclusive events.

21. **What is a Venn diagram? How would two mutually exclusive events (A and B) be illustrated in Venn format?**

    In a Venn diagram, events are represented as simple geometric figures, with overlapping areas of events represented by intersections and unions of the figures. Two mutually exclusive events (A and B) are represented in a Venn diagram by two nonintersecting areas. As may be seen in Figure 14-1, events A and B are mutually exclusive because there is no overlap. The probability of their occurring simultaneously, therefore, = 0.

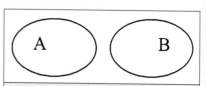

Figure 14-1. Venn diagram representing two mutually exclusive events (A and B).

22. **How would the intersection of two mutually exclusive events be represented in mathematic notation?**

$$P(A \text{ and } B) \text{ or } P(A \cap B) = 0.$$

    P(A ∩ B) is the event that both A and B occur simultaneously and is read as "the intersection of events A and B."

23. **What does the Venn diagram look like if the events are not mutually exclusive?**

    If two events A and B are not mutually exclusive, the Venn diagram circles will intersect at some point (*see* Fig. 14-2). The intersecting area is represented by the equation P(A and B) = P(A and B occur together) or P(A ∩ B) > 0.

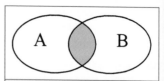

Figure 14-2. Venn diagram of two events (A and B) that are not mutually exclusive.

24. **What is the multiplicative (i.e., product) rule?**

The multiplicative rule applies when calculating the probability of at least two *independent events* occurring *together*. The multiplicative rule states the following:

$$P(A \text{ and } B) = P(A) \times P(B)$$

where $P(A \text{ and } B)$ represents the probability of both A and B occurring together and $P(A)$ and $P(B)$ represent the independent probabilities of A and B, respectively.

If A and B are independent events, then the following equation applies:

$$P(A \text{ and } B) \text{ or } P(A \cap B) = P(A) \times P(B)$$

25. **What is the probability of rolling two successive 5s in a row with a single unbiased die?**

Here is an opportunity to use the product rule. We have established that successive rolls of a die are independent events, and we know that we can expect to roll a 5 one out of every six times, on average. Given that A (the first roll) and B (the second roll) are independent events, then $P(A \text{ and } B)$ or $P(A \cap B) = P(A) \times P(B)$.

$$
\begin{aligned}
P(\text{rolling two fives}) &= P(\text{rolling 5}) \times P(\text{rolling 5}) \\
&= 1/6 \times 1/6 \\
&= 1/36 \\
&= 0.028
\end{aligned}
$$

26. **Can the product rule be used to determine the probability of more than two events occurring?**

Yes. As long as the events are truly independent, there is no limit to the number of events that can be considered.

27. **According to a national survey, 63% of voting Americans prefer presidential candidate A. If three voters in the United States are chosen at random, what is the probability that all three will prefer candidate A?**

For multiple events $(A_1, A_2, A_3, ...A_X)$, if $A_1, A_2, A_3, ...A_X$ are mutually independent, then $P(A_1 \text{ and } A_2 \text{ and } A_3 \text{ and}, ...A_X) = P(A_1) \times P(A_2) \times P(A_3) ... P(A_X)$. Therefore, the probability of all three voters preferring candidate A:

$$
\begin{aligned}
&= P(A) \times P(A) \times P(A) \\
&= 0.63 \times 0.63 \times 0.63 \\
&= 0.25
\end{aligned}
$$

28. **Assume that you are given only the probabilities of being male (0.35) and being elderly (0.60) from the results in question 3. Using these figures, what is the probability that a patient diagnosed with disease Y will be male *and* elderly [P(male, elderly)], assuming that being male and being elderly are mutually independent?**

$$
\begin{aligned}
P(\text{male and elderly}) &= P(\text{male}) \times P(\text{elderly}) \\
&= 350/1000 \times 600/1000 \\
&= 0.21
\end{aligned}
$$

29. **In the previous question, is it correct to assume that being male and being elderly are independent events?**

Probably not, but if you are given only the marginal probabilities of each event, there is no way to tell for certain. Beware: false claims of statistic support often treat events as independent when, in fact, they are not.

30. **How then do we calculate the probability of both events taking place when the events are not independent?**

When the events are not independent, we can use a special form of the product rule that takes into account the lack of independence:

$$P(A \text{ and } B) = P(A \mid B) P(B)$$

The conditional probability of A given B is multiplied by the marginal probability of B. Importantly, and usefully, this rule can also be written as:

$$P(A \text{ and } B) = P(B \mid A) P(A)$$

31. **Now, assuming that being male and being elderly are *not* independent events and that data are available, how would we calculate the probability that a patient diagnosed with disease Y will be male *and* elderly [P(male, elderly)]?**

First, consult Table 14-1 for the appropriate data related to elderly and male patients, and fill in the appropriate numbers:

$$P(A \text{ and } B) = P(A \mid B) P(B)$$
$$P(\text{male, elderly}) = P(\text{male} \mid \text{elderly}) P(\text{elderly})$$
$$= (200/600) \times (0.6)$$
$$= 0.33 \times 0.6$$
$$= 0.20$$

32. **Prove that P(A and B) = P(A | B) P(B) = P(B | A) P(A)**

Using the same data, we find

$$P(\text{male, elderly}) = P(\text{elderly} \mid \text{male}) P(\text{male})$$
$$= (200/350) \times (350/100)$$
$$= 0.571 \times 0.35$$
$$= 0.20$$

33. **Based on the previous work, are being male and elderly independent events?**

No. When the assumption of independence was made, the probability of being male and elderly was 0.21, but when actual data were used, the probability was in fact 0.20. Though unequal, these results show that the assumption of independence was actually reasonable for a ballpark estimate for this particular data set; the conditional probability of being elderly given male was 0.57, not far off from the marginal probability of being elderly in the entire population (0.6). However, do not extrapolate this example as a generality. Often, incorrectly making the assumption of independence will give results that are grossly in error.

34. **What is the additive rule?**

The additive rule is used to calculate the probability that one of at least two events will occur. The additive rule states that $P(A \text{ or } B) = P(A) + P(B) - P(A \text{ and } B)$. This rule is illustrated in a Venn diagram in Figure 14-3. For mutually exclusive events (*see* Fig. 14-1), this equation reduces to $P(A \text{ or } B) = P(A) + P(B)$, because, by definition, $P(A \text{ and } B) = 0$ for mutual exclusivity to occur.

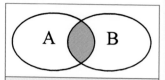

Figure 14-3. Venn diagram of the additive rule for two events (A and B) that are not mutually exclusive.

KEY POINTS: PROBABILITY

1. Probability quantifies the likelihood of occurrence of event A over unlimited trials.

2. The standard equation for probability is P(event) = A/N.

3. The additive rule states that P(A *or* B) = P(A) + P(B) − P(A and B).

4. The multiplicative rule for independent events states that P(A *and* B) = P(A) × P(B).

5. If two events are not independent, a special form of the multiplicative rule can be used, as follows: P(A and B) = P(A | B) P(B) = P(B | A) P(A).

---

35. **Using the spreadsheet in Table 14-1, what is the probability that a patient diagnosed with disease Y will be female *or* elderly?**
    Gender and elderly age grouping are *not* mutually exclusive; therefore, using the additive rule, the equation P(A *or* B) = P(A) + P(B) − P(A and B) applies as follows:

    $$P(\text{female or elderly}) = P(\text{female}) + P(\text{elderly}) - P(\text{female and elderly})$$
    $$= 650/1000 + 600/1000 - 400/1000$$
    $$= 0.85$$

36. **This is rather confusing. Is there an algorithmic method of approaching the probability of more than one event?**
    See Figure 14-4.

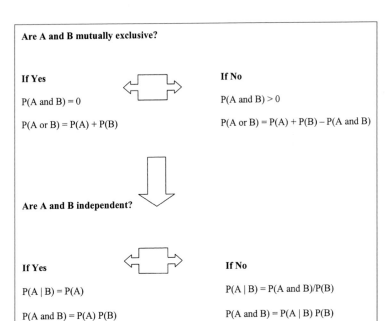

Figure 14-4. Algorithmic method of approaching the probability of more than one event.

SAMPLING

37. What is sampling?
Sampling is a technique used by researchers to collect measurements from a sample population with the goal of making inferences about an overall target population.

38. Why conduct sampling?
Economic and logistic constraints often make it difficult, expensive, or even destructive (depending on the type of research in question) to collect measurements in an entire target population, forcing researchers to collect data from a small segment of a population for extrapolation to the target population. When making generalizations to the target population based on sample results, however, we must understand the inherent limitations of sampling.

39. What is a target population?
The target population is the group of subjects, objects, measurements, or events that the sample is meant to represent.

40. What is the most important characteristic of a good sample?
The sample must represent the population from which it is taken if generalizations about the target population will be made from the sample data analysis.

41. Explain sampling error.
Sampling carries an inherent likelihood of sampling error (i.e., the difference between a measured characteristic in the sample and in the target population). In reality, this error can rarely be determined because the true target population measurement is not generally known.

42. What are the main causes of error in sampling?
Sampling error is known to have two major causes: selection bias and random variation. Selection bias error is caused by using a sample population with measurement characteristics that are not representative of the target population. Random variation error is measurement error attributable simply to chance.

43. Which type of error can be minimized by proper study design and sampling technique?
Selection bias can be minimized by using a randomized selection process. Random variation error is "random," attributed to chance, and thus not controllable.

44. How is sampling performed?
Numerous mechanisms for sampling are available, including the following:
- Simple random sampling
- Stratified random sampling (i.e., random sampling of each group after division into heterogeneous groups)
- Clustered random sampling (i.e., random sampling of groups after division into homogeneous groups)
- Systematic random sampling (e.g., sampling every 10th, 20th, etc.)

45. Why is randomization desired in the sample selection?
Randomization will help to ensure that the sample is representative of the overall target population. The researcher should keep in mind that the sampling process—not the sample itself—determines randomness. Ideally, random sampling eliminates bias, leaving random variation as the only possible source of error, with the magnitude of that error determined by the size of the sample and the heterogeneity of the population.

KEY POINTS: SAMPLING

1. Sampling allows a researcher to make inferences about a target population by using only a portion of the population, known as a sample.

2. A good sample must be representative of the characteristics of the target population.

3. Sampling error is caused by selection bias and random variation.

4. Randomization is a tool to minimize selection bias.

5. Estimation of sample size is performed before conducting a study to assess the feasibility and constraints of performing the study.

46. Why is the determination of an adequate sample size important in planning a study?

Sample size determination is a critical step in research planning because sample size is often a key factor in determining time and funding necessary to complete a study. Furthermore, an inadequate sample size may lead to a lack of statistic significance in the resultant data.

47. What factors affect sample size?

Consider the simplest possible formula for sample size determination, the paired *t*-test:

$$N = z_\alpha^2 \times (s)^2/(d)^2$$

where d represents the mean difference that was observed, $(s)^2$ represents the variance of the mean difference, and z_α represents the required level of significance. Rosner describes four major factors affecting sample size when this formula is used:

- Sample size increases as variance increases.
- Sample size increases as the significance level is made smaller (i.e., α decreases).
- Sample size increases as the required power increases (i.e., $1-\beta$ increases).
- Sample size decreases as the absolute value of the distance between the null and alternative means increases.

WEBSITE

http://www.amstat.org/sections/epi/SIE_Home.htm

BIBLIOGRAPHY

1. Morton RF, Hebel JR, McCarter RJ: A Study Guide to Epidemiology and Biostatistics, 5th ed. Gaithersburg, MD, Aspen Publications, 2001, pp 51–69.

2. Rosner B: Fundamentals of Biostatistics, 5th ed. Pacific Grove, Duxbury, 2000, pp 45–77.

3. Schwartz BS, Mitchell CS, Weaver VM: Occupational Medicine Board Review Course Notes, ACOEM 1:210–214, 2000.

CHAPTER 15

CHARACTERISTICS OF DIAGNOSTIC TESTS

Ward L. Reed, MD, MPH

1. **What is a test?**
   This may seem like a slightly basic and ridiculous question, but you need to keep your mind open as to what a test is. Many readers of this book have a fixed idea of a "test." They consider it as something that is ordered on a slip of paper or computer screen, after which blood is drawn, a radiologic or other procedure is performed, and, at some point in the future, the results of the test are returned, either by computer or another slip of paper.

   Although much of the information in this chapter applies directly to this model, expand your view of a "test." *A test is any procedure that determines a state, quantity, or amount of a subject.*

2. **What are some examples of tests that one typically does not consider a "test?"**
   The act of interviewing a new patient is a test. Taking vital signs is a series of tests. Physical examination is also a series of tests. Looking at a traffic light to see what color it is can be viewed as a test. The performance of all of these tests can be analyzed. For example, you may be comfortable discussing the sensitivity of a blood test for a certain disease, but the sensitivity and specificity of the presence of rales in pneumonia are at least as important.

3. **How are different types of tests classified?**
   Usually, tests are described according to how the results are reported. Results are considered quantitative, semiqualitative, or qualitative.

4. **Describe quantitative tests.**
   Quantitative tests give numeric results. Usually, quantitative test results are considered as continuous variables in statistical considerations. In the examples given above, blood pressure, temperature, and serum cholesterol are examples of quantitative testing. The results of a quantitative test must always be expressed in specific units and not just as a number or result.

5. **Describe qualitative tests.**
   Qualitative tests give binary (i.e., dichotomous) results. Qualitative tests are considered as categorical variables in statistical considerations. Categorical data are characteristics with discrete values or types. Typical examples of qualitative results are dead or alive, male or female, presence or absence of a rash, and the like.

6. **Describe semiquantitative tests.**
   Semiquantitative tests can be viewed as multiple-level qualitative tests. They are almost always considered as categorical variables in statistical considerations. Examples of semiqualitative results are categories of hurricanes (1–5), grading of reflexes (0–4+), and clinic evaluation of strength (0–5). Although these results are ranked, one must take care not to assume that the differences are linear. For example, the wind speeds in a level 5 hurricane are not five times greater than those in a level 1 hurricane.

KEY POINTS: TYPES OF TESTS

1. Quantitative test: gives results as a number, treated as continuous variable.

2. Qualitative test: gives results as a yes or no, treated as categorical variable.

3. Semiqualitative test: gives results (usually) as a number but is a ranking that cannot be considered linear. Although they look like continuous variables, cannot be treated as such in biostatistics.

7. Can quantitative test results be converted to categorical outcomes?
They can and often are. Although the results of quantitative tests are given as numeric answers (e.g., LDL cholesterol of 145±8 mg/dL), they are usually presented as a qualitative result (e.g., normal or abnormal; or positive or negative). The performance of a quantitative test, when converted to categorical outcomes, depends on the inherent performance of the test (determined by its standard deviation, which, in turn, is determined by technical factors of the test) and at what point the test is considered "abnormal" or "positive." The same test will have differing performance depending on where the line is placed between normal and abnormal. Often, an "indeterminate" range is given for an outcome, indicating that a clinic decision cannot be made on the basis of that test result alone.

8. What is the difference between accuracy and precision?
Accuracy and precision are terms that are usually applied to quantitative tests. The two terms are often used interchangeably by the lay public, but they have specific meanings in the field of statistics. *Accuracy* is the ability to produce a result that is very close to the accepted standard. This result may be a mean of widely disparate results, but if the average is very close to the accepted answer, the test is considered "accurate." *Precision* refers to the ability to reproduce the same result consistently (Fig. 15-1). This result may not be that close to the accepted answer, but the results are reproducible.

9. Give examples of accuracy and precision.
Imagine two scales on which you are going to weigh yourself. As a scientist, you know to perform multiple trials of a measurement and then average the results. Here are the results:
- Scale 1: 68 kg, 70 kg, 75 kg, 72 kg, 65 kg
- Scale 2: 73.5 kg, 73 kg, 72.5 kg, 73 kg, 73 kg

You determine later, using the gold standard, that your correct weight is 70 kg. Scale 1 is accurate (the mean is 70 kg), but scale 2 is precise (the mean is 73 kg; standard deviation [SD] = 0.35). This example also illustrates that a given test may be useful, even if inaccurate. If you are starting an exercise program to lose weight, you would be more likely to choose scale 2; even though its answer is 3 kg from the accepted standard, it will give more consistent results, allowing interval changes to be more apparent. Figure 15-2 may be used to illustrate qualitatively the distribution of many trials using the two scales.

10. What determines when a "positive" test is "positive"?
There are two ways that the normal range for a test can be determined: the population-based approach and the condition-based approach.

11. Explain the population-based approach to determining the normal range.
A population-based approach usually assumes that any person with a value greater than 2 SDs from the mean, assuming a normal distribution, is abnormal. A large amount of data is collected

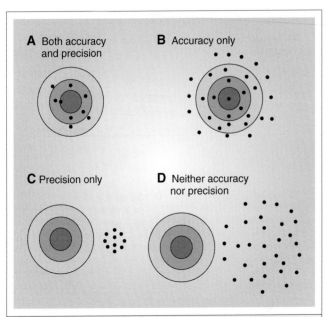

Figure 15-1. Possible combinations of accuracy and precision in describing a contiguous variable, using a target and bullet holes to demonstrate the concepts. (From Jekel JF, Katz DL, Elmore JG: Epidemiology, Biostatistics, and Preventive Medicine, 2nd ed. Philadelphia, W.B. Saunders, 2001.)

on normal people (i.e., those without apparent disease), and the normal range is determined from those data. Note that, by its very nature, this method will result in an "abnormal" test for 5% of a normal population.

12. **When can the population-based approach be used?**
The above method works only when the distribution of the characteristic in the population is normally distributed. Often the characteristic is not normally distributed. In this case, a frequency distribution table should be used to determine where the upper and lower 2.5% lie.

13. **Are abnormal test results always indicative of disease?**
An abnormal test does not necessarily mean disease. Many tests in a standard screening panel have normal ranges, determined using the population approach. As a result, many times "abnormal" does not mean "diseased"; it may simply mean "different." In fact, if the tests are assumed to be independent, a battery of 20 is more likely than not to return an abnormal test. The probability of an abnormal test is 5% (0.05); thus, the probability of a normal test is 0.95. The probability of 20 normal tests in a row is 0.95^{20}, or 0.36. Thus, the probability that a completely normal (nondiseased) individual will have one test in a panel of 20 is 0.64, or more likely than not.

14. **How is "abnormal" determined using the condition-based method?**
The condition- or disease-based method attempts to determine (usually by large epidemiologic studies) what value is associated with a given condition. For example, according to the most recent Joint Nation Commission on Heart Disease (JNC 7), the normal range for systolic blood pressure (as defined by no excess risk of cardiovascular disease) is 115 mmHg or less. At this level,

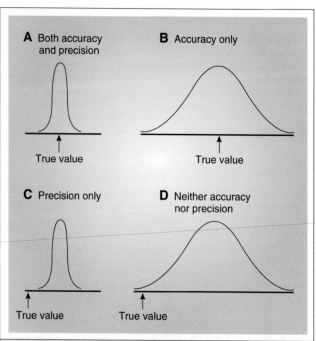

Figure 15-2. Possible combinations of accuracy and precision in describing a continuous variable. The x-axis is a range of values, with the arrow indicating the true value. The curves are the probability distributions of observed values. (From Jekel JF, Katz DL, Elmore JG: Epidemiology, Biostatistics, and Preventive Medicine, 2nd ed. Philadelphia, W.B. Saunders, 2001.)

significantly more than 5% of the population have an abnormal value, which points out that "normal" often changes. Thirty years ago, physicians accepted elevated blood pressures in the elderly as "normal aging," although the same patients are now routinely treated.

Chobanian AV, Bakris GL, Black HR, et al: Seventh Report of the Joint National Committee on Prevention, Detection, Evaluation, and Treatment of High Blood Pressure. Hypertension 42(6):1206–1252, 2004.

15. **What is meant by the term "gold standard"? What implications does it have?**
The performance of all tests must have some benchmark with which to compare the results of a new test. That benchmark is usually referred to as the gold standard. The gold standard is usually the definitive test for any disease state or condition. For example, although there are many types of rapid assays for streptococcal pharyngitis, the gold standard is still the identification of beta-hemolytic streptococcus on throat culture. The gold standard test is often not used routinely because it may be expensive (e.g., a magnetic resonance imaging [MRI] scan), invasive (e.g., a biopsy), dangerous, or sometimes all of the above (e.g., cardiac catheterization).

16. **How golden are the gold standards?**
Most gold standards are alloys, and some of them have been proven to be iron pyrite (fool's gold). Because of difficulties in easily confirming negative diagnoses in some cases, inappropriate or inadequate control groups (conditions thought to be consistent with disease later shown

to be normal variants) and the lack of established clinic standards for a disease both contribute to inaccurate gold standards. As a result, a new test will not appear to perform any better than the gold standard, even though, in reality, it may be superior.

17. **Why are two-by-two (2 × 2) tables important? What is in them?**
Two-by-two tables are, in some respects, the very essence of epidemiology and biostatistics, as well as other disciplines. (It has been said that "you are nobody in psychology unless you have your name attached to your own 2 × 2 table.") The typical setup of a 2 × 2 table is shown in Table 15-1. The disease state is put on one axis, and the tested state is placed on the other. The values outside the box are called *marginals*. (See m1–m4 in the table.) It is important to realize that *there is no standard way to set up a 2 × 2 table*. The information in Table 15-1 could just as easily have been presented as it is in Table 15-2.

TABLE 15-1.   SET UP OF TWO-BY-TWO TABLE

	Disease Positive	Disease Negative	
Test Positive	a	b	m3
Test Negative	c	d	m4
	m1	m2	

TABLE 15-2.   ALTERNATE SET UP OF TWO-BY-TWO TABLE

	Test Positive	Test Negative
Disease Positive	a	c
Disease Negative	b	d

18. **Define true positive and true negative.**
A *true positive* is the instance in which a diagnostic test correctly determines the positive state of the tested individual. A *true negative* is the instance in which a test correctly identifies a nondiseased (or negative) individual as being negative. The true blocks are indicated in Table 15-3.

19. **Define false negative and false positive.**
False negatives are instances when a test has incorrectly classified a positive individual as negative. *False positives* occur when a negative individual is incorrectly identified as being positive. The false blocks are also indicated in Table 15-3.

TABLE 15-3.   TRUE AND FALSE BLOCKS IN A TWO-BYTTWO TABLE

	Disease Positive	Disease Negative
Test Positive	True Positive	False Positive
Test Negative	False Negative	True Negative

20. How is sensitivity defined?

Sensitivity is defined as the fraction of people with the disease or condition who are correctly identified as positive. Looking again at the archetypical 2 × 2 table, the sensitivity is calculated as

$$\frac{\text{No. with condition testing positive}}{\text{Total number with condition}}$$

The actual calculation from Table 15-4 would be a/(a + c), or a/m1. Readers are encouraged to learn the general equation, not the shortened a/(a + c) version. As indicated previously, because the presentation of the data can change, the simplified formula may not always work.

TABLE 15-4. TWO-BY-TWO TABLE FOR CALCULATION OF SENSITIVITY AND SPECIFICITY

	Disease Positive	Disease Negative	
Test Positive	a	b	m3
Test Negative	c	d	m4
	m1	m2	

KEY POINTS: 2 × 2 TABLES

1. 2 × 2 tables are the standard way to present data on test performance.

2. True positives are people with the condition who test positive.

3. True negatives are people without the condition who test negative.

4. False positives are people without the condition who test positive.

5. False negatives are people with the condition who test negative.

21. Give an example of a calculation for sensitivity.

A set of diagnostic criteria was tested against accepted clinic practice, and the results are shown in Table 15-5. The sensitivity in this case would be 29/(29 + 26) = 0.527, or 52.7%. This result is considered fairly poor.

TABLE 15-5. TEST CRITERIA VERSUS CLINIC PRACTICE

	Clinically Positive	Clinically Negative
Test Positive	29	3
Test Negative	26	28

22. How is specificity defined?

As sensitivity deals with those who test positive, specificity deals with those who test negative. Specificity is defined as the fraction of tested people identified as negative. The general formula is

$$\frac{\text{No. without condition testing negative}}{\text{Total number without condition}}$$

The general calculation from Table 15-4 would be $d/(b + d)$, or d/m^2.

23. **Give an example of a specificity calculation.**
    Using the data from testing diagnostic criteria in Table 15-5, the calculated sensitivity would be $28/(28 + 3) = 0.903$, or 90.3%.

24. **What is the relationship between specificity and the rate of false positives?**
    Because specificity indicates how well a diagnostic test identifies true negatives, intuitively we expect that there is a relationship between those identified correctly as negative and those truly negative who are falsely identified as positive. In fact, the false-positive rate can be calculated directly from the given specificity. Generally, true positives (TP) + false positives (FP) = all positive tests. The false-positive rate (FPR) can also be calculated from the specificity since true negatives (TN) + false positives (FP) = all disease negatives (DN). Dividing by DN and rearranging, we obtain $1 - \text{TN/DN} = \text{FP/DN}$. Thankfully, this equation simplifies to

$$1 - \text{specificity} = \text{FPR}$$

25. **How does sensitivity relate to the rate of false negatives?**
    As sensitivity and false-positive rate are related, so are specificity and false negatives related. The general formula for false-negative rate (FNR) is

$$\text{FNR} = \frac{\text{No. with the condition testing negative}}{\text{Total number with condition}}$$

From the general 2×2 table, the calculation would be $b/(b + d)$. Similar to specificity and the false-positive rate, the false-negative rate is more easily calculated as

$$1 - \text{sensitivity} = \text{FNR}$$

26. **What is positive predicted value?**
    Positive predictive value (PPV) is the proportion of a tested population with a positive test who actually had the disease or condition in question. The denominator includes the true positives and the false positives. PPV is dependent on the performance of the test in the tested population and the prevalence of the condition in the tested population.

27. **What is the formula for positive predictive value?**
    The general equation for PPV is

$$\frac{\text{True positives}}{\text{All positives}}$$

or

$$\frac{\text{True positives}}{\text{True positives + false positives}}$$

28. **In the case of the data presented in Table 15-5, what is the PPV?**

$$\text{PPV} = 29/(29 + 3) = 90.1\%$$

29. **What is negative predicted value?**
    Negative predictive value (NPV) is the proportion of tested population with a negative test who actually did not have the disease or condition in question. The denominator includes the true negatives and the false negatives. NPV also depends on both performance of the test and prevalence of the condition of interest.

30. **What is the general equation for negative predicted value?**
The general equation for NPV is

$$\frac{\text{True negatives}}{\text{All negatives}}$$

or

$$\frac{\text{True negatives}}{\text{True negatives + false negatives}}$$

KEY POINTS: SENSITIVITY, SPECIFICITY, AND PREDICTIVE VALUE

1. Sensitivity = TP/(TP + FN)

2. Specificity = TN/(TN + FP)

3. Positive predictive value = TP/(TP + FP)

4. Negative predictive value = TN/(TN + FN)

5. Predictive value depends on the performance of the test, combined with the prevalence of the condition in the tested population.

31. **In the case of the data presented in Table 15-5, what is the negative predictive value?**
As mentioned, the PPV is 29/(29 + 3) or 90.1%, a seemingly useful result. The NPV is 28/(28 + 26) or 51.8%, which is only slightly better than the flip of a coin. Remember that predictive values of a given test are a function of the performance of the test as well as the prevalence of the studied condition in the population being studied.

32. **Can the predictive value of a test change if the test performance does not?**
Yes. The terms "PPV" and "NPV" usually refer to data taken from test performance. The performance of the test and the predictive value of the test will vary with the prevalence of the disease in the test population.

33. **Give an example of changing disease prevalence.**
A researcher has discovered a marker in blood that she believes will be useful in screening for inflammatory bowel disease (IBD). The initial tests are done on consecutive patients in the waiting area of a gastroenterology (GI) clinic at a large tertiary care facility. The hypothetic results are shown in Table 15-6. These data yield a sensitivity of 95%, a specificity of 98%, PPV of 92%, and NPV of 98%.

Now imagine that the experiment is repeated, except that the study population is taken from the waiting area of a blood donor center. The results may look like Table 15-7. These data yield a sensitivity of 100%, a specificity of 96%, PPV of 33%, and NPV of 100%. Note that the change in the tested population completely alters the usefulness of the test. By altering the prevalence of the disease in the tested population from 30% in the GI clinic to 2% in the general population, there is a huge difference in the predictive values of the tests. The difference in the sensitivity and specificity is due to rounding errors; in these examples it is not possible to have a fraction of a person. It is possible, however, to have differences in test performance in different populations. Differences in stages of disease and characteristics of the population can (and often do) change the performance of the test itself. This shows the influence of prevalence on predictive value. It also stresses the importance of knowing from where data on test performance come.

TABLE 15-6.   RESULTS OF SCREENING TEST FOR IBD IN GI CLINIC

	Clinically Positive	Clinically Negative
Test Positive	57	5
Test Negative	3	135

TABLE 15-7.   RESULTS OF SCREENING TEST FOR IBD IN BLOOD DONOR CENTER

	Clinically Positive	Clinically Negative
Test Positive	10	20
Test Negative	0	470

34. What is pretest probability?
Pretest probability is the baseline likelihood that a given condition exists in the population in question. Most often it is prevalence of a condition in the studied population, although this can be altered, given other factors.

35. Why is pretest probability important in evaluating diagnostic tests?
Sensitivity and specificity are important factors in evaluating the performance of diagnostic tests, but they are not the only factors. As important, and sometimes more important, is the frequency of the condition in the tested population. The pretest probability is determined in a number of ways. The easiest is to consider the frequency of the condition in the general population, namely the incidence or prevalence of the condition. Ideally, the prevalence in the specific population would be known (e.g., the prevalence of coronary artery disease in 55-year-old, left-handed, diabetic plumbers experiencing increasing bouts of atypical chest pain), but often an ideal level of detail is not available. In such cases, pretest clinic perception is often substituted.

36. What is Bayes' theorem?
Bayes' theorem is named for Thomas Bayes (1702–1761), a Nonconformist minister and amateur mathematician who lived in England. Elected Fellow of the Royal Society in 1742 (mainly for a defense of Newton's calculus), his most important contribution was his theory of probability, which was published posthumously in 1764.

Bayes' theorem predicts the probability of event A given event B. The general form of Bayes' theorem is

$$P(A \mid B) = \frac{P(B \mid A)P(A)}{P(B \mid A)P(A) + P(B \mid {\sim}A)P({\sim}A)}$$

The notation $P(A)$ is read as "the probability of A." The notation $P(A \mid B)$ is read as "the probability of A given B." The notation $P(B \mid {\sim}A)$ is read as "the probability of B given 'not A.'" In order to figure out the probability of A given B, we need to know the probability of B given A, the probability of A, the probability of B given "not A," and the probability of "not A." Bayes' theorem can be used for such diverse applications as determining the probability of making the third traffic light after getting through the first two, to determining what is spam (unsolicited commercial e-mail) in your inbox.

37. **What does Bayes' theorem have to do with diagnostic testing?**
Bayes' theorem is often used as the basis for determining PPV and NPV. Positive and negative predictive value can be calculated when the raw data from a test trial are presented, but such data are not usually presented. Using Bayes' theorem, the PPV is

$$P(\text{disease} \mid +\text{test}) = \frac{P(\text{test} + \mid \text{disease})P(\text{disease})}{P(\text{test}+ \mid \text{disease})P(\text{disease}) + P(\text{test}+ \mid \sim\text{disease})P(\sim\text{disease})}$$

38. **That is rather complicated. Is there a simpler form of Bayes' theorem?**
The equation is simpler if you realize that most of the terms are actually easily obtainable. The definition of sensitivity is P(test+ | disease). The P(disease) is either the prevalence of the condition or the clinic pretest probability. The P(test+ | ~disease) is the same as 1 – specificity. The probability of no disease is either 1 – prevalence or 1 – pretest probability. Simplifying the equation, we have

$$P(\text{disease} \mid +\text{test}) = \frac{\text{Sens} \times \text{prevalence}}{\text{Sens} \times \text{prevalence} + (1 - \text{spec})(1 - \text{prevalence})}$$

This equation is most often cited as the calculation for the predictive value of a positive test.

39. **Is there also a simplified equation for the negative predictive value?**
Likewise, the predictive value of a negative test can be simplified to

$$P(\text{disease} \mid -\text{test}) = \frac{\text{Spec} \times (1 - \text{prevalence})}{\text{Spec} \times (1 - \text{prevalence}) + (1 - \text{sens})(\text{prevalence})}$$

40. **Show how Bayes' theorem can be used in the clinic setting.**
A second-year medical student reads about visceral trypanosomiasis (i.e., sleeping sickness). He realizes that he is often very sleepy, gets headaches, and has some sore joints. He thinks some of his lymph nodes are enlarged. He comes to the conclusion that somehow he has contracted African trypanasomiasis (sleeping sickness). He talks a lab technician into running an enzyme-linked immunosorbent assay (ELISA) blood test for trypanosomiasis, and the result is elevated. Should he next call the Centers for Disease Control and Prevention (CDC) for treatment?
Assume that the sensitivity and specificity of the test are both 90% and that the prevalence in second-year medical students in the United States is 1 in 5,000,000.

Posttest probability = $(0.90)(2 \times 10^{-7})/ [(0.90)(2 \times 10^{7})+(0.10)(1 - 2 \times 10^{-7})] = 1.8 \times 10^{-6}$

KEY POINTS: BAYES' THEOREM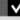

1. Bayes' theorem calculates probabilities of events after an observed event.

2. The most useful form of Bayes' theorem in diagnostic testing is for positive predictive value, as follows:

$$P(\text{disease} \mid +\text{test}) = \frac{\text{Sens} \times \text{prevalence}}{\text{Sens} \times \text{prevalence} + (1 - \text{spec})(1 - \text{prevalence})}$$

41. **What is a likelihood ratio?**
A likelihood ratio is a clinic tool used to combine the sensitivity and specificity in a more user-friendly way than Bayes' theorem. It is a measure of the odds of results in a diseased and a nondiseased group. By multiplying the pretest odds by the likelihood ratio, the posttest (i.e., posterior) odds can be obtained. Note that the likelihood ratio uses odds rather than

probabilities, like Bayes' theorem. Likelihood ratios are an expression of the degree to which a positive or negative test influences the odds of disease after the test. The closer the likelihood ratio is to 1, the less useful is the test.

42. **How is the likelihood ratio calculated?**
There are forms of likelihood ratio (LR) for both a positive test and a negative test, as follows:

$$LR(positive) = \frac{Sensitivity}{1 - specificity}$$

$$LR(negative) = \frac{1 - sensitivity}{Specificity}$$

43. **A new type of rapid MRI examination for shoulder labrum tears has a sensitivity of 0.85 and a specificity of 0.90. What are the LR (positive) and LR (negative)?**
- LR+ = 0.85/(1 − 0.90) = 8.5
- LR− = (1 − 0.85)/0.90 = 0.167
The farther away from 1 a test's likelihood ratio is, the more useful that test is considered.

44. **How is the likelihood ratio used?**
The prior probability (i.e., prevalence or a priori pretest probability) is converted to odds form, as necessary. The prior odds are multiplied by the appropriate form of the likelihood ratio and are then converted back to probability. One of the useful aspects of the likelihood ratio is that multiple tests can be evaluated with one set of calculations by stringing likelihood ratios together.

45. **A team physician for a minor league baseball team is evaluating a pitcher for shoulder pain. Based on the pitcher's history and a physical examination, the physician believes that the player has a shoulder labrum tear that will require surgical correction. He then sends the patient for the rapid MRI examination referenced in question 43. What is the probability that the pitcher has an operable shoulder lesion after a positive test?**
- Step 1. Convert to odds: odds = probability/(1 − probability) = 0.60/(1 − 0.60) = 1.5
- Step 2. Multiply by LR+: posterior odds = LR × prior odds = 8.5 × 1.5 = 12.75
- Step 3. Convert back to probability: probability = odds/(1 + odds) = 12.75/13.75 = 0.92

46. **After learning the results of the tests, the pitcher (who is averse to surgery) wants more tests. The physician reluctantly arranges another study that has a sensitivity of 0.8 and a specificity of 0.95 and yields a negative result. What is the posttest probability after the second test? Assume that the tests are independent.**
We can begin with the posterior odds of the previous problem, 12.75.
- Step 1. Calculate LR− as follows: LR− = (1 − sensitivity)/specificity = (1 − 0.8)/0.95 = 0.21
- Step 2. Multiply odds by LR−: 12.75 × 0.21 = 2.68
- Step 3. Convert to probability: Probability = odds/(1 + odds) = 2.68/3.68 = 0.72
    Note that the second confirmatory test done to rule out a diagnosis only lowered the probability of that diagnosis from 0.92 to 0.72. The diagnosis is still more likely than not.

47. **What is an ROC curve?**
The ROC curve stands for *receiver operator characteristic* curve. It is used to graphically represent the response of a test to the variation of a positive level. When a test is reported as a quantitative result, the value that is positive may be varied. There is almost always some kind of trade-off between sensitivity and specificity. A level may be chosen that results in identification of almost all diseased individuals, but this level will usually result in a large proportion of false positives and, thus, a low specificity. A level at which almost all nondiseased individuals are

correctly identified will result in very low sensitivity (i.e., true-positive rate). The ROC curve graphically demonstrates how the altered levels change the sensitivity and specificity.

KEY POINTS: LIKELIHOOD RATIOS (LRS)

1. Likelihood ratios (LRs) calculate similar data using odds ratios and can be used serially.

2. $LR(positive) = \dfrac{Sensitivity}{1 - Specificity}$

3. Posterior odds = initial odds $\times LR_1 \times LR_2 ... LR_x$

4. $LR(negative) = \dfrac{1 - Sensitivity}{Specificity}$

5. The LR calculation assumes that the tests are independent (i.e., the results of one have no effect on the results the others).

---

48. **How is an ROC curve drawn?**
The ROC curve is a plot of the false-positive rate (i.e., 1 − specificity) versus the sensitivity. The data from the varied levels are determined, and then the plot is drawn. The data from a trial of fasting plasma glucose for the diagnosis of gestational diabetes mellitus are shown in Table 15-8. There are always two fixed points on an ROC curve: 0,0 and 1,1. These points represent the extremes, at which all nondiseased (100% specificity, 0% sensitivity) or all diseased (0% sensitivity, 100% specificity) cases are identified. The plot is seen in Figure 15-3. This is a typical ROC curve. The more a curve reaches the upper left of the plot, the better a diagnostic test is said to perform.

Perucchi D, Fischer U, Spinas G, et al: Using fasting plasma glucose concentrations to screen for gestational diabetes mellitus: Prospective population-based study. BMJ 319:812–815, 1999.

TABLE 15-8. PLASMA GLUCOSE FOR DIAGNOSIS OF GESTATIONAL DIABETES					
Glucose level (mmol/L)	5.2	5.0	4.8	4.6	4.4
Sensitivity	0.55	0.62	0.81	0.92	1.0
Specificity	0.96	0.88	0.76	0.60	0.39

49. **What is a "good" ROC curve?**
ROC curves are evaluated by the area under the curve. A "perfect" ROC curve would yield an area of 1. A totally useless test would give a straight line with a slope of 1 and, thus, an area of 0.5. For simple curves with few data points, areas are calculated by a geometric method. For more complex curves with many data points, a fairly complex nonparametric statistical method is used. A rule of thumb for evaluating ROC curves is as follows:
- 0.90–1.00 = excellent
- 0.80–0.90 = good
- 0.70–0.80 = fair
- 0.60–0.70 = poor
- < 0.60 = worthless

ROC curves may also be used to choose where to place the point at which a test is considered positive. Figure 15-4 graphically illustrates the usefulness of given ROC curves. The points in the upper left of the curve have the best balance of sensitivity and specificity.

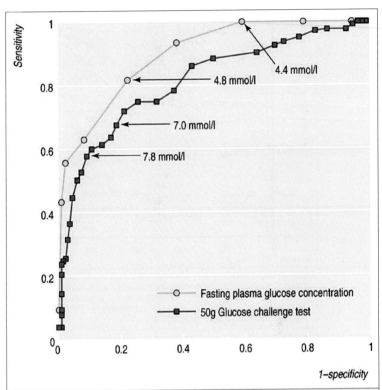

Figure 15-3. Receiver operating characteristic (ROC) curve for fasting glucose concentration as a test for diagnosing gestational diabetes mellitus. (From Perruchini D, Fischer U, Spinas GA, et al: Using fasting plasma glucose concentration to screen for gestational diabetes mellitus: Prospective population-based study. BMJ 319[7213]:812–815, 1999, with permission.)

50. **What is the difference between serial and parallel testing?**
In clinic medicine there are two strategies for multiple testing. In *serial testing,* the results of test 1 are considered before test 2, the results of test 2 are considered before test 3, and so on. In order to be considered positive, all tests in the series must be positive. In *parallel testing,* all tests are considered independently, and any positive is considered a positive.

KEY POINTS: RECEIVER OPERATOR CHARACTERISTICS (ROC) CURVES

1. The performance of a test will change depending upon where a positive is placed.

2. The ROC curve is drawn by plotting the false-positive rate (i.e., 1 – specificity) on the x-axis versus sensitivity on the y-axis.

3. A useless ROC curve is a straight line with a slope of 1. The more the curve bends to the upper left of the graph, the better the test is said to perform.

4. The performance of a test is measured by area under the curve: 1 is perfect and 0.5 is useless.

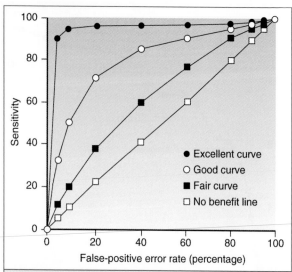

Figure 15-4. Examples of receiver operating characteristic (ROC) curves for four tests. The uppermost curve is the best of the four. (From Jekel JF, Katz DL, Elmore JG: Epidemiology, Biostatistics, and Preventive Medicine, 2nd ed. Philadelphia, W.B. Saunders, 2001.)

51. How does one decide which strategy is appropriate?

Serial testing is useful when false positives are undesirable, such as when treatment is highly invasive or toxic. *Parallel testing* is useful when rapid diagnosis is necessary and a missed diagnosis is undesirable.

52. When are serial and parallel testing strategies used?

Serial testing produces in an overall highly specific but insensitive strategy, whereas parallel testing yields a sensitive but not specific strategy. For example, in the emergency department, multiple tests are ordered in a parallel fashion when a patient presents with the chief complaint of chest pain. If any one of the tests shows positive results, including an S-T segment elevation on an electrocardiogram (ECG), an elevated serum troponin level, or signs of left-sided heart failure on chest radiograph, the patient is deemed to be having a myocardial infarction and is treated accordingly. Conversely, a surgical oncologist will not remove a colon on the basis of a positive test for blood in the stool (a common screening test for colon cancer with easy administration and low cost); surgery requires confirmatory tests, which are done serially.

53. Why is independence important in testing?

Independence in testing affects how tests are interpreted. In considering multiple serial tests, it is usually assumed that the outcomes of each test are not dependent on the others. Thus, the final odds of disease in a series of tests will be

$$\text{Odds(final)} = \text{odds(initial)} \times LR_1 \times LR_2 \times LR_3...LR_x$$

In reality, however, tests are often not independent; a false-positive result on one may predispose to a false-positive (or false-negative) result on another. Many tests may, in function, be looking for the same thing or may be done in the same way; thus, the weakness of one may well be the weakness of another. Ideally, we want test performance data related to the series of tests; unfortunately, such data usually are not available.

54. How is agreement among different raters measured?
Determinations of categorical data, such as interpretation of radiologic studies, depend on the judgment of the rater (e.g., judging the presence of infarcts on MRI or the presence of malignant cells in a biopsy). For validity of results, the same study is usually examined by multiple evaluators. Cohen's kappa (i.e., the kappa test) is used to quantitate the degree of agreement among individual raters, taking into account the agreement caused by chance. The test is reported on a scale from −1 to +1.

KEY POINTS: PARALLEL AND SERIAL TESTING

1. Parallel testing involves a series of tests done simultaneously: with any one positive test, the entire series is considered positive.

2. Serial testing involves a series of tests done sequentially: all must be positive to be considered positive.

3. Parallel testing results in a sensitive but nonspecific strategy; serial testing is specific but not sensitive.

55. What is a good kappa score?
A kappa of less than 0.6 is usually considered unacceptable, whereas a kappa greater than 0.80 is excellent. A weighted kappa can be used wherein some disagreements are considered worse than others (e.g., normal vs. highly malignant biopsy).

56. How is the kappa statistic calculated?
The most common version of the kappa statistic, Cohen's kappa, is calculated by comparing expected versus observed agreement. Using the 2×2 format in Table 15-9, the calculations are as follows:
- P(observed agreement) = $(a + d)/N$
- P(expected) = $[(f1 \times g1) + (f2 \times g2)]/N^2$
- Kappa = $[P(observed) - P(expected)]/[1 - P(expected)]$

TABLE 15-9. DATA NEEDED FOR KAPPA CALCULATION

		Observer 1		
		Yes	No	
Observer 2	Yes	a	b	g1
	No	c	d	g2
		f1	f2	N

57. Give an example of kappa calculation.
Two 6-year-olds at a park are asked to decide which animals are squirrels. The tabulation of their results is shown in Table 15-10.

- P(observed) = (31 + 41)/84 = 0.77
- P(expected) = (43 × 38 + 41 × 46)/(84)^2 = 0.50
- Kappa = (0.77 − 0.50)/(1 − 0.5) = 0.54

In this case, the kappa is 0.54; the agreement between the two six-year-olds is not very good. Possibly there may be an error in perception (i.e., one of the children needs glasses) or training (i.e., misidentification of cats, chipmunks, field mice, and other small mammals), but in any event, conclusions based on the data from these observers would be rather suspect.

TABLE 15–10. EXAMPLE OF DATA FOR KAPPA CALCULATION

		Observer 1		
		Squirrel	Not Squirrel	
Observer 2	Squirrel	31	7	38
	Not Squirrel	12	34	46
		43	41	84

58. Can kappa be calculated for more than two observers?
The above calculation of Cohen's kappa is the simplest possible, with two observers and two outcomes. When multiple observers and multiple outcomes are possible, the calculation becomes far more complex and is almost always done by computer.

It is worth noting that the kappa statistic is not universally recognized as a gold standard evaluation. The exact interpretation of the statistic is subject to disagreement, and the weighting values (when used) are arbitrary and, thus, are subject to bias.

WEBSITE

http://www.apha.org/public_health/epidemiology.htm

BIBLIOGRAPHY

1. Chobanian AV, Bakris GL, Black HR, et al: Seventh Report of the Joint National Committee on Prevention, Detection, Evaluation, and Treatment of High Blood Pressure. Hypertension 42(6):1206–1252, 2004.

2. Jekel JF, Katz DL, Elmoe JG: Epidemiology, Biostatistics, and Preventive Medicine, 2nd ed. Philadelphia, W.B. Saunders, 2001.

3. Perucchi D, Fischer U, Spinas G, et al: Using fasting plasma glucose concentrations to screen for gestational diabetes mellitus: Prospective population-based study. BMJ 319:812–815, 1999.

CHAPTER 16

THE STUDENT'S *t*-DISTRIBUTION AND STUDENT'S *t*-TEST

Philip D. Parks, MD, MPH

1. **How are the *t*-distribution and *t*-test used? What types of data can be interpreted?**
   The *t*-distribution and the Student's *t*-test are used for inference about a population mean using small samples (<30) when the data are derived from a simple random sample. In this chapter's examples, it is assumed that when the *t*-distribution and Student's *t*-test are being used, the simple random sample is taken from an approximately normal population and the population standard deviation (σ) is unknown.

2. **For which student is the Student's *t*-test named?**
   Copyright laws established by his employer (Guinness Brewery) prevented William Gossett (1876–1937) from naming one of the most commonly used statistical tests after himself. Instead of naming this useful tool Gossett's test, he used the pseudonym "Student" when he wrote his description in 1908 of the *t*-distribution and what he called the Student's *t*-Test. As the Guinness Brewery quality control engineer, Gossett used his new *t*-procedures to compare batches of stout and solidified his employment by helping the brewery produce the cheapest and best beer possible.

3. **Why not use the *z*-distribution (i.e., normal distribution)?**
   Inference procedures for means associated with the normal curve (*z*-procedures) are appropriate only when the standard deviation of the population (σ) is known. Typically, we would expect σ to be unknown; thus, in medical research, the *t*-procedures are generally utilized. For sample sizes greater than about 30, however, the *z*-distribution and the *t*-distribution are nearly identical.

4. **For what other sampling designs are *t*-procedures appropriate?**
   We also use *t*-procedures to compare the responses to two treatments in two independent groups or in one group of subjects at two different times. The comparison is made by applying the *t*-procedures to the observed differences. If we wish to compare responses to two treatments or to compare means of two populations, we need independent simple random samples from (ideally) approximately normal populations in which the means and standard deviations are unknown. These procedures are robust as long as the population distributions have similar shapes and the data include no strong outliers.

5. **How is a *t*-test about μ performed?**
   Several variations of the *t*-test are covered throughout this chapter, but the general approach is as follows:
   1. State the default condition for μ giving the hypothesized value (in H_0) and the claim about μ for which we are gathering evidence (H_a).
   2. (a) Determine the critical ratio (the difference between the sample mean and the hypothesized population mean divided by the standard error [SE] of the sample mean).
      (b) Compare the critical ratio to the appropriate *t*-value in the table.
   3. Reject H_0 or do not reject H_0.
   4. Write the conclusion.

6. **What is the paired *t*-test?**
   In medical literature, studies often compare the effects of medications on patients. For example, if we want to investigate the effect of cholesterol-lowering medications, we may compare the

data of a patient on medication to that of the same patient when not on medication. Using this matched pair (also known as the before-and-after method), a patient serves as his own control. The paired *t*-test considers variation from only one sample group, whereas the two-sample *t*-test considers variation from two independent groups. Therefore, using the paired *t*-test is a good way to focus on variation that is determined by the effect of the intervention or changes over time in the same subject.

7. **Which new variable is used in the paired *t*-test?**
   In order to perform the paired *t*-test, a new variable (d) is used. The variable represents the difference between the data before and after the intervention was introduced to the subjects being studied. We perform the *t*-test on the difference data. The variable $\bar{d}$ represents the mean observed difference between the initial (i.e., baseline) and final values (after the intervention was imposed) or, generally for paired data, the mean of the difference data.

8. **What do the results of *t*-tests tell us?**
   Gossett's model, the Student's *t*-distribution, is used for interference (hypothesis testing and calculating confidence intervals) about population means; in other words, to determine (for one sample) whether or not the difference between the sample mean and the population mean exceeds the difference that would be expected by chance alone, from random sampling. The test is used to assess whether difference is statistically significant.

9. **What are some variations of applications of the *t*-test?**
   There are variations of the Student's *t*-test: the one-tailed test and the two-tailed test (also known as one-sided and two-sided tests). For example, the one-tailed test is used when testing whether μ is greater or less than the hypothesized population mean, μ_0, but the researcher is only testing the "greater" or the "less than"—not the possibility that μ could be either one. A two-tailed test is used for testing μ not equal μ_0; in other words, it could be either greater or less than.

10. **What is the standard error of the sample mean?**
    The standard error of the sample mean (SE) is the ratio of the sample standard deviation to the $\sqrt{sample\ size}$ and is used in the calculation of the critical ratio *(t)* for a *t*-test. Just as the standard deviation describes the variability of observations, the standard error measures the variability of means. The standard error can be thought of loosely as the standard deviation of the sample means, and "error" is a traditional statistical term for chance variation.

11. **How is the standard error calculated for a single sample?**
    For one sample, the standard error can be calculated using the sample standard deviation if the sample size is known. Standard Error $= \dfrac{s}{\sqrt{n}} = \sqrt{\dfrac{s^2}{n}}$. From this calculation, we observe that as the sample size (n) increases, the standard error decreases.

12. **What are degrees of freedom?**
    The degrees of freedom are dependent upon and calculated from the sample size for a one-sample calculation. In a distribution, the degrees of freedom are the number of parameters that may be independently varied and are used to make adjustments for the sample size.

13. **How is the degree of freedom calculated for a single sample or for matched pairs?**
    For a one sample or a matched-pairs design, the degrees of freedom (df) is defined as one less than the number of observations n(df = n − 1); in other words, only n − 1 observations can vary freely. Thus, if the sample size is 15, the degrees of freedom (df) is 14.

14. **How are degrees of freedom calculated for two independent samples?**

As long as population variances are equal, the degrees of freedom for the two independent samples is the sum of the degrees of freedom for each sample. Sometimes you see this written as $df = (n_1 - 1) + (n_2 - 1) = n_1 + n_2 - 2$. For example, if one sample is of size 14 and the other sample is of size 17, the df (for the two-sample model) $= (14 - 1) + (17 - 1) = 29$.

15. **Why is the degrees of freedom important?**

The degrees of freedom is used along with the critical ratio and Gosset's model, the Student's t-distribution, to approximate the likelihood (i.e., probability) that a value as extreme as the critical ratio occurs by chance alone. As the degrees of freedom increases, the t-curve becomes similar in appearance to the normal or z-curve. (*See* Fig. 16-1.)

Moore DS: The Basic Practice of Statistics, 2nd ed. New York, W.H. Freeman & Company, 2000.

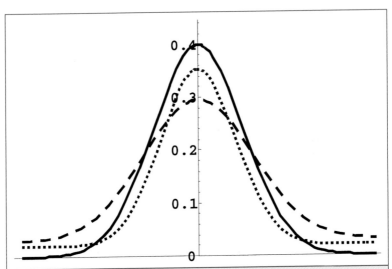

Figure 16-1. Degrees of freedom. Unbroken line = standard normal distribution; dotted line = t-distribution with 9 degrees of freedom; and dashed line = t-distribution with 4 degrees of freedom.

16. **How do results of procedures using the t-distribution differ from those using the z-distribution?**

When using the t-distribution model versus the normal model (i.e., z-distribution), the confidence intervals will be slightly wider and the p-values slightly larger. The t-distribution is different from the normal distribution because the standard deviation is dependent upon sample size. When sample sizes are 30 or larger, the t-distribution and z-distribution are essentially identical.

As the sample size increases, the t-curve approaches the normal curve with increasing similarity. This occurs because the sample standard deviation (s) more precisely estimates the population standard deviation (σ). Therefore, with large samples, replacing σ with s causes minor variation.

17. **What are critical ratios?**

The different variations of t-tests support conclusions about population means by calculating a ratio called the *critical ratio*. This critical ratio is compared with values in a statistic table (e.g., a table of t-values) for the observed degrees of freedom. The statistic tables are included in Appendixes A and B of this book. A critical ratio for means is defined as the difference in the sample and population means divided by the standard error of the sample mean.

$$\text{Critical Ratio} = \frac{\text{Difference in the sample mean and population mean}}{\text{Standard Error of the sample mean}}$$

Or written with standard statistical symbols, $t = \dfrac{\overline{x} - \mu 0}{s/\sqrt{n}}$ [$\overline{x}$ = mean of the sample;

$\mu 0$ = hypothesized mean of the population; s = standard deviation of the sample; n = sample size]

18. **How do we calculate critical ratios for a one-sample test about the mean?**
Suppose we gather the following information for a one-sample test: the sample mean is 10, the population mean is 9.6, and the sample standard deviation is 1 for a sample of size 16. Then

$$\text{CriticalRatio} = t = \frac{\overline{x} - \mu 0}{s/\sqrt{n}} = \frac{10 - 9.6}{1/\sqrt{16}} = \frac{0.4}{0.25} = 1.6$$

19. **How do we calculate critical ratios for a test for matched-pairs data?**
Suppose we gather data for a matched-pairs design. So we have two sets of data that are matched pairs. For example, data set 1 is collected from nine subjects before an intervention and data set 2 is collected from the same nine subjects after the intervention. The first step is to calculate the difference data (d) and then apply the one-sample procedures to this data set. We keep in mind that f for the difference data will always be 0 if there is *no* difference in the matched-pairs data. Suppose that the sample mean (of the difference data) is −1.2 and that the sample standard deviation (of the difference data) is 1 for a sample of size 9. Then

$$\text{CriticalRatio}_d = t_d = \frac{\overline{d} - \mu 0}{s_d/\sqrt{n}} = \frac{-1.2 - 0}{1/\sqrt{9}} = \frac{-1.2}{1/3} = -3.6$$

The d subscripts are a reminder that these calculations are about the difference data for the matched-pairs data. In the paired *t*-test, the mean is only calculated once. Therefore, only one degree of freedom is lost.

20. **How do we calculate critical ratios for a test for two-sample data?**
For a two-sample test, the samples must be independent and each sample should be from an underlying normal population for which the population standard deviations are unknown.

$$t = (\overline{x}_1 - \overline{x}_2) - (\mu_1 - \mu_2)$$

Notice that we subscript the quantities associated with sample 1 and 2 with the

appropriate subscripts. Sometimes $\mu_1 - \mu_2 = 0$, and the calculation becomes $t = \dfrac{(\overline{x}_1 - \overline{x}_2)}{SED(\overline{x}_1 - \overline{x}_2)}$.

21. **How do you calculate the standard error of the difference (SED) and the degrees of freedom when comparing two independent samples?**
The calculations for the two-sample situation are very cumbersome and are usually supported by technology. We have two choices for the calculations for $SED(\overline{x}_1 - \overline{x}_2)$ and *df.* (1) nonpooled (when it is known that the underlying populations do not have equal variances), and (2) pooled (when we are willing to assume that the underlying populations have equal variances).

$$\text{For non-pooled, } SED(\overline{x}_1 - \overline{x}_2) = \sqrt{\frac{s_1^2}{n_1} + \frac{s_2^2}{n_2}} \text{ and}$$

$$df = \frac{\left(\dfrac{s_1^2}{n_1} + \dfrac{s_2^2}{n_2}\right)^2}{\dfrac{1}{n_1 - 1}\left(\dfrac{s_1^2}{n_1}\right)^2 + \dfrac{1}{n_2 - 1}\left(\dfrac{s_2^2}{n_2}\right)^2} \text{ (round this value downward to the next integer)}$$

For pooled, we first estimate the common variance $s_p^2 = \dfrac{(n_1 - 1)\,s_1^2 + (n_2 - 1)\,s_2^2}{n_1 + n_2 - 2}$

$$SED_{pooled}(\bar{x}_1 - \bar{x}_2) = \sqrt{\frac{s_p^2}{n_1} + \frac{s_p^2}{n_2}} \text{ and } df = (n_1 - 1) + (n_2 - 1) = n_1 + n_2 - 2$$

22. **What does the size of the critical ratio indicate?**

In each case, we look up the critical ratio in the appropriate statistical table to determine the value of p (i.e., the probability that the observed mean is due to chance alone). The larger the critical ratio (and the smaller the p), the more likely the difference between the sample and the hypothesized population mean (or means) is not due to random variation and the difference is statistically significant. In general, in the medical literature, if the p-value is ≤ 0.05, the difference is considered significant. The degrees of freedom is used in the tables to adjust the critical ratios for the sample size. When using the tables, consider the absolute value of the critical ratio (e.g., if $t = -2.50$, calculate probabilities using $t = 2.50$).

23. **What are the one-tailed and two-tailed *t*-tests?**

When we perform tests of significance, we start with a null hypothesis (H_0), the default statement about our hypothesized population parameter. The test will assess the strength of the evidence against H_0. The alternative hypothesis (H_a) indicates the effect for which we hope to find supporting evidence. H_a may be one-sided (for example, $H_a = \mu > 0$ or $H_a = \mu < 0$) or two-sided (for example, H_a: $\mu \neq 0$). One-sided alternative hypotheses establish interest in extreme effects in one direction or another, whereas two-sided tests address whether the parameter of interest differs from some value.

24. **How do we complete a one-sample *t*-test?**

Our situation is as follows: we have 10 healthy female patients ages 30–35 who never exercise. Table 16-1 gives each patient's most recent hip bone density reading (mg/cm^2). Do these data provide conclusive evidence at the 5% level of significance that healthy female patients ages 30–35 who never exercise have bone density results lower than the average of 945 mg/cm^2?

1. For H_0 $\mu = 945$ and for H_a $\mu < 945$ [a left-tailed test—one-sided]

2. $t = \dfrac{\bar{x} - \mu}{s/\sqrt{n}} = t \sim \dfrac{940.6 - 945}{11.66/\sqrt{10}} \sim -1.1933$ and $df = 10 - 1 = 9$

   From Table 16-2, for the area in the left tail of the *t*-distribution to be less than 5% with 9 degrees of freedom, our critical ratio must be ≤ -1.833. The value of t is -1.1933, which is >-1.8333 (i.e., further from 0).

3. We cannot reject H_0.

4. Based on these data, we do not have evidence at the 5% level of significance to conclude that healthy female patients ages 30–35 who never exercise have bone density results lower than the average of 945 mg/cm^2.

TABLE 16-1.	MOST RECENT HIP BONE DENSITY READING (MG/CM^2) IN 10 PATIENTS									
Patient	1	2	3	4	5	6	7	8	9	10
Bone density	948	940	950	920	936	952	958	934	940	928

25. **How do we complete a matched-pairs *t*-test?**

Consider the following example: we have 13 patients whom we have been treating with cholesterol-lowering drugs. Table 16-3 gives the total cholesterol level before treatment and the total cholesterol

TABLE 16-2.   SIGNIFICANCE LEVEL FOR ONE-DIRECTION STUDENT *t*-TEST[*]

df	.10	.05	.025	.01	.005	.000
1	3.078	6.314	12.706	31.821	63.657	636.619
2	1.886	2.920	4.303	6.965	9.925	31.598
3	1.638	2.353	3.182	4.541	5.841	12.941
4	1.533	2.132	2.776	3.747	4.604	8.610
5	1.476	2.015	2.571	3.365	4.032	6.859
6	1.440	1.943	2.447	3.143	3.707	5.959
7	1.415	1.895	2.365	2.998	3.499	5.405
8	1.397	1.860	2.306	2.896	3.355	5.041
9	1.383	**1.833**[†]	2.262	2.821	3.250	4.781
10	1.372	1.812	2.228	2.764	3.169	4.587
11	1.363	1.796	2.201	2.718	3.106	4.437
12	1.356	**1.782**[‡]	2.179	2.681	3.055	4.318
13	1.350	1.771	2.160	2.650	3.012	4.221
14	1.345	1.761	2.145	2.624	2.977	4.140
15	1.341	1.753	2.131	2.602	2.947	4.073
16	1.337	1.746	2.120	2.583	2.921	4.015
17	1.333	1.740	2.110	2.567	2.898	3.965
18	1.330	1.734	2.101	2.552	2.878	3.922
19	1.328	1.729	2.093	2.539	2.861	3.883
20	1.325	1.725	2.086	2.528	2.845	3.850
21	1.323	1.721	**2.080**[§]	2.518	2.831	3.819
22	1.321	1.717	2.074	2.508	2.819	3.792
23	1.319	1.714	2.069	2.500	2.807	3.767
24	1.318	1.711	2.064	2.492	2.797	3.745
25	1.316	1.708	2.060	2.485	2.787	3.725
26	1.315	1.706	2.056	2.479	2.779	3.707
27	1.314	1.703	2.052	2.473	2.771	3.690
28	1.313	1.701	2.048	2.467	2.763	3.674
29	1.311	1.699	2.045	2.462	2.756	3.659
30	1.310	1.697	2.042	2.457	2.750	3.646
40	1.303	1.684	2.021	2.423	2.704	3.551
60	1.296	1.671	2.000	2.390	2.660	3.460
120	1.289	1.658	1.980	2.358	2.617	3.373
χ	1.282	1.645	1.960	2.326	2.576	3.291

[*]For a calculated *t*, if |t| (absolute value of t) is greater than the value shown, reject the null hypothesis.
[†]See question 24.
[‡]See question 25.
[§]See question 27.

level after 60 days of medication. Do these data provide evidence at the 5% level of significance to conclude that the medication produced a reduction in cholesterol level?

To complete a matched-pairs test, we must first calculate the difference data (Table 16-4). A "reduction in total cholesterol level" means the difference that we calculate (before and after) is greater than zero.

1. For H_0 $\mu_d = 0$ and for H_a $\mu_d > 0$ [a right-tailed test—one-sided]

2. $t_d = \dfrac{\bar{d} - \mu}{s_d / \sqrt{n}} \sim \dfrac{24.62 - 0}{14.93 / \sqrt{13}} \sim 5.9457$ and $df = 13 - 1 = 12$

From Table 16-2, for the area in the left tail of the *t*-distribution to be less than 5% for 12 degrees of freedom, our critical ratio must be ≥ 1.782. The value of *t* is 5.9457, which is ≥ 1.782

3. We strongly reject H_0.

4. Based on these data, we have strong evidence at the 5% level of significance to conclude that the medication produced a reduction in total cholesterol level.

TABLE 16-3. TOTAL CHOLESTEROL BEFORE AND AFTER TREATMENT

Patient	1	2	3	4	5	6	7	8	9	10	11	12	13
Before treatment	220	240	190	210	250	230	240	250	230	225	180	200	230
After treatment	198	199	182	200	228	215	200	190	200	208	160	175	220

TABLE 16-4. CALCULATION OF THE DIFFERENCE DATA

Patient	1	2	3	4	5	6	7	8	9	10	11	12	13
Difference data: Before–After	22	41	8	10	22	15	40	60	30	17	20	25	10

26. **How do we complete a two-sample *t*-test?**

Consider the following example: we want to test the effectiveness of a new headache medication. We randomly assign 12 headache patients to an experimental group that takes the medication for 1 month and 12 headache patients to a control group that takes a placebo for 1 month. The patients return and complete the Headache Assessment Survey. Results are given in Table 16-5. Do these data provide evidence at the 5% level of significance to conclude that results in the Headache Assessment Survey are different for the experiment versus the control groups?

We will not assume that the underlying populations (i.e., Headache Assessment Survey Results for all patients who take the medication and the Headache Assessment Survey Results for all patients who take the placebo) have equal variances. Thus, we will complete the non-pooled calculations.

1. For H_0, $\mu_E = \mu_C$ and for H_a, $\mu_E \neq \mu_C$ [a two-tailed test—two-sided]

2. $t = \dfrac{(\bar{x}_E - \bar{x}_C)}{SED(\bar{x}_E - \bar{x}_C)}$ and $SED(\bar{x}_E - \bar{x}_C) = \sqrt{\dfrac{s_E^2}{n_E} + \dfrac{s_C^2}{n_C}} = \sim \sqrt{\dfrac{18.56^2}{12} + \dfrac{16.64^2}{12}} \sim 7.196$

Therefore, $t = \dfrac{(\overline{X}_E - \overline{X}_C)}{SED(\overline{X}_E - \overline{X}_C)} \approx \dfrac{58.67 - 48.5}{7.196} = 1.413$ and

$$df = \dfrac{\left(\dfrac{s_1^2}{n_1} + \dfrac{s_2^2}{n_2}\right)^2}{\dfrac{1}{n_1 - 1}\left(\dfrac{s_1^2}{n_1}\right)^2 + \dfrac{1}{n_2 - 1}\left(\dfrac{s_2^2}{n_2}\right)^2} \approx \dfrac{\left(\dfrac{18.56^2}{12} + \dfrac{16.64^2}{12}\right)^2}{\dfrac{1}{12 - 1}\left(\dfrac{18.56^2}{12}\right)^2 + \dfrac{1}{12 - 1}\left(\dfrac{16.64^2}{12}\right)^2} \approx \dfrac{2681.196}{123.314} \approx 21.74$$

Therefore, rounding down, use df = 21. From Table 16-6, for the area in both tails of the *t*-distribution to be less than 5%, our critical ratio must be ≥2.080. The value of *t* is 1.413, which is ≤2.080.

3. We cannot reject H_0.
4. Based on these data, we do not have evidence at the 5% level of significance to conclude that results in the Headache Assessment Survey are different for the experiment group versus the control group.

TABLE 16-5.   HEADACHE SURVEY SCORES

Experiment group	64	56	36	55	20	70	80	77	68	60	78	40
Control group	33	50	45	80	22	40	64	50	72	44	34	48

27. **Can one use a one-tailed table to calculate a *p*-value for a two-tailed test, as in the previous question ?**
Yes. However, sometimes only one-tailed tables are available. Because the *t*-distribution is symmetric about zero, one can easily perform two-tailed calculations using one-tailed tables. The trick is that you must divide the desired probability by 2 to account for both tails. In question 26, for example, by using a two-tailed table we found that our critical ratio must by greater than 2.080 for at least 95% probability of being correct in rejecting the null hypothesis. Using a one-tailed table, we would choose 0.025 as the "tail probability," because both tails were considered. This "tail probability" would be 0.025 × 2 = 0.05, the value used directly on a two-tailed table. Now using df = 21 and probability value of 0.025 on a one-tailed table, we find that the critical ratio must be greater than 2.080—precisely the result obtained from the two-tailed table. (*See* Table 16-2.)

28. **What are confidence intervals?**
The confidence interval (CI) is an interval for capturing a population parameter (e.g., the mean or μ) with endpoints calculated from the data as follows: $\overline{x}$ ± (confidence coefficient)(SE). The confidence coefficient is chosen to give an estimate that will result in a given level of confidence that the parameter is within the boundaries of the interval. For example, for a 95% CI, the confidence coefficient is the *t*-value, taken from the appropriate table, which separates the central 95% of the distribution from the tail area.

29. **How do we calculate a 95% confidence interval?**
Suppose that we have an appropriate set of data for which n = 18, $\overline{X}$ = 42, and s = 6.3. Let us create a 95% CI for μ, the true mean of the population from which the data set was taken. *Note:* Since df = 18 – 1 = 17, the critical ratio (t_C) = 2.110 for a two-tailed test (*see* Table 16-2).

$$\overline{x} \pm (\text{95\% confidence coefficient})(SE) = 42 \pm 2.110\,(6.3/\sqrt{18}) \Rightarrow$$

$$42 - 2.110\,(6.3/\sqrt{18}) \approx 38.87 \text{ and } 42 + 2.110\,(6.3/\sqrt{18}) \approx 45.13$$

TABLE 16-6.	SIGNIFICANCE LEVEL FOR TWO-DIRECTION STUDENT *t*-TEST*					
df	.20	.10	.05	.02	.01	.001
1	3.078	6.314	12.706	31.821	63.657	636.619
2	1.886	2.920	4.303	6.965	9.925	31.598
3	1.638	2.353	3.182	4.541	5.841	12.941
4	1.533	2.132	2.776	3.747	4.604	8.610
5	1.476	2.015	2.571	3.365	4.032	6.859
6	1.440	1.943	2.447	3.143	3.707	5.959
7	1.415	1.895	2.365	2.998	3.499	5.405
8	1.397	1.860	2.306	2.896	3.355	5.041
9	1.383	1.833	2.262	2.821	3.250	4.781
10	1.372	1.812	2.228	2.764	3.169	4.587
11	1.363	1.796	2.201	2.718	3.106	4.437
12	1.356	1.782	2.179	2.681	3.055	4.318
13	1.350	1.771	2.160	2.650	3.012	4.221
14	1.345	1.761	2.145	2.624	2.977	4.140
15	1.341	1.753	2.131	2.602	2.947	4.073
16	1.337	1.746	2.120	2.583	2.921	4.015
17	1.333	1.740	2.110	2.567	2.898	3.965
18	1.330	1.734	2.101	2.552	2.878	3.922
19	1.328	1.729	2.093	2.539	2.861	3.883
20	1.325	1.725	2.086	2.528	2.845	3.850
21	1.323	1.721	**2.080**†	2.518	2.831	3.819
22	1.321	1.717	2.074	2.508	2.819	3.792
23	1.319	1.714	2.069	2.500	2.807	3.767
24	1.318	1.711	2.064	2.492	2.797	3.745
25	1.316	1.708	2.060	2.485	2.787	3.725
26	1.315	1.706	2.056	2.479	2.779	3.707
27	1.314	1.703	2.052	2.473	2.771	3.690
28	1.313	1.701	2.048	2.467	2.763	3.674
29	1.311	1.699	2.045	2.462	2.756	3.659
30	1.310	1.697	2.042	2.457	2.750	3.646
40	1.303	1.684	2.021	2.423	2.704	3.551
60	1.296	1.671	2.000	2.390	2.660	3.460
120	1.289	1.658	1.980	2.358	2.617	3.373
χ	1.282	1.645	1.960	2.326	2.576	3.291

*For a calculated *t*, if |t| (absolute value of t) is greater than the value shown, reject the null hypothesis.
†See question 24.

Therefore, the 95% CI is (38.87, 45.13), and we can say that if we collected similar data many times and calculated 95% CIs from the data, 95% of the confidence intervals would contain the true population mean.

30. **How do we know whether *t* or *z* should be used?**

Using principles of statistic inference, we can draw generalized conclusions about a population using data from a random sample. The procedures for constructing confidence intervals about μ (i.e., population mean) with σ (i.e., population standard deviation) unknown are similar to when σ is known. However, s is used instead of σ, and *t* (for the *t*-distribution) is used instead of *z* (for the normal distribution). Therefore, when σ is known, *z*-intervals are constructed and when σ is unknown, *t*-intervals are constructed.

KEY POINTS: THE *t*-DISTRIBUTION AND STUDENT'S *t*-TEST

1. When utilizing the *t*-test procedures, the assumptions are that (1) the sample is a simple random sample from an approximately normally distributed population; (2) the population standard deviation is unknown; and (3) one or both sample sizes are less than 30.

2. Use the *t*-test to compare a sample mean and a population mean, two independent samples, or the same sample at two different times (often before and after treatment).

3. The *t*-distribution is similar to the normal distribution in three ways: (1) it is symmetric about 0; (2) it is bell-shaped; and (3) it is single-peaked.

4. The *t*-distribution differs from the normal distribution in that (1) the *t*-distribution has larger tails than the normal distribution (i.e., the *t*-distribution has more probability in the tails); (2) a greater number of degrees of freedom (df) means smaller tails (therefore, the larger the df, the closer to the normal distribution); and (3) a smaller df means larger tails.

5. For samples greater than 30, the *t*-distribution is nearly identical to the normal distribution (i.e., *z*-distribution).

31. **How does the width of a confidence interval vary and affect its usefulness?**

The usefulness of the interval is determined by its width (i.e., the difference between the upper and lower endpoints). Wide intervals do not provide us with precise information about the location of the true population mean. Also, wide intervals may indicate that collecting more data may help in describing something definite about the given parameter. Narrow intervals provide us with better information about the location of the population mean.

32. **How does the range of the confidence interval differ with changes in the confidence level?**

If the sample size n remains the same, decreasing the confidence level of an interval decreases the width of the confidence interval, and increasing the confidence level of an interval increases its precision. Generally, confidence levels are chosen to be 95%, but confidence intervals of 90%, 99%, and 99.9% can be considered.

33. **What is the sum of squares?**

The sum of squares (SS) or total sum of squares (TSS) is defined as the sum of the squares of the standard deviations. SS and TSS are usually associated with analysis of variance (ANOVA), a specific method for analyzing variation among multiple groups.

34. **What is ANOVA? When is it used?**

    It is a statistics test of significance designed to determine whether a significant difference exists among multiple sample means. The F statistic relates the ratio of the variance occurring between the means to the variance that occurs within groups themselves. The larger the F statistic, the more significant the result. SS is used to calculate the ANOVA F statistic.

35. **What is chi-square? When is it used?**

    A chi-square test is a test of statistical significance that does not specifically test a population parameter (like the mean). A chi-square test is used in two situations:

    - Goodness of fit: this hypothesis test addresses the issue of whether the distribution of a given data set in categories "fits" a uniform distribution of the data.
    - Independence: this hypothesis test addresses the issue of whether the categories in a two-way contingency table are related.

WEBSITE

http://www.csm.ornl.gov

BIBLIOGRAPHY

1. Altman DG: Practical Statistics for Medical Research. Boca Raton, FL, CRC Press, 1990.
2. Bland M: An Introduction to Medical Statistics, 3rd ed. Oxford, Oxford University Press, 2000.
3. Dawson BK: Basic and Clinical Biostatistics, 3rd ed. New York, McGraw-Hill/Appleton & Lange, 2000.
4. Moore DS: The Basic Practice of Statistics, 2nd ed. New York, W.H. Freeman & Company, 2000.
5. "Student" (W.S. Gosset): The probable error of a mean. Biometrika 6(1):1–25, 1908.
6. Zar JH: Biostatistical Analysis, 4th ed. Princeton, NJ, Prentice Hall, 1999.

CHAPTER 17

BIVARIATE ANALYSIS

Moore H. Jan, MD, MPH

1. **What is bivariate analysis?**
   Univariate analysis involves collecting and analyzing data on one variable. In bivariate analysis, we extend this process to *two* variables.

2. **Why is bivariate analysis performed?**
   Bivariate analysis is performed when one believes there may be some association between the two variables. Typically, one is searching for a relationship indicating a risk factor (an independent variable) and a health outcome (a dependent variable). This chapter examines some of the methods employed in bivariate analysis.

3. **Does a found association indicate a causal relationship?**
   No. Finding an association is merely the first step toward supporting a cause-and-effect relationship between two variables.

4. **What methods are used to determine associations between variables?**
   Several statistic methods are used to identify associations. To a large degree, the methods that we can use depend on the characteristics of the data.

5. **What is a good first question one might ask when choosing a statistic method?**
   A good first question is whether the data are quantitative or qualitative. Quantitative data are numeric, with some sense of rank or order. Qualitative data are categoric, such as gender (e.g., male or female) or race.

6. **Can quantitative data be further grouped?**
   Yes. Quantitative data can be further grouped into continuous versus discrete data.

7. **Are there restrictions on the values that a continuous variable may be assigned?**
   There are no restrictions on the value that a continuous variable can assume. A variable designated for human height is a clear example of a quantitative continuous variable. Any value along the continuum of potential weights may be the assigned value.

8. **What is discrete about discrete data?**
   Discrete data can assume only certain values. For example, a variable designated as the number of nevi on a person can assume only discrete integer values (e.g., 0, 1, 2, 3,...).

9. **Does it matter how the data are presented when deciding the best methods of analysis?**
   Yes. In bivariate data analysis, one must consider the properties of each variable because each may have different characteristics. For example, a data set composed of individual blood pressure measurements and ages in years represents a pairing of continuous and discrete data. The selection of the best analysis tool is dependent on both variables.

10. **What are paired data?**
    In paired data, the value of one variable is assumed to be associated with the value of the other, usually because they represent data on a single entity or object (e.g., an individual). Whether or not the data are paired also restricts the choice of bivariate statistic methods.

11. **When dealing with continuous data, are there any considerations with respect to our analysis?**
    Yes. For continuous data, we must consider the distribution of the data and ask, "Can the assumption of a normal distribution be made?"

12. **What are parametric tests?**
    Many tests assume normality (i.e., the data follow a normal or binomial distribution), and these are called parametric tests. Examples of parametric tests include Pearson's correlation and linear regression tests.

13. **What if the assumption of normality cannot be made for the data set?**
    Tests that make no assumption of normality are termed *nonparametric*. Examples of nonparametric tests include the Wilcoxon signed rank test, the Mann-Whitney *U* test, the Kruskal-Wallis test, and the McNemar test. Deciding whether or not to use a parametric versus a nonparametric test can be difficult. Sometimes tests for normality can help.

14. **List methods commonly used to analyze quantitative continuous data.**
    - Scatterplots
    - Pearson's correlation
    - Simple linear regression
    - Spearman's rank correlation (nonparametric)
    - Wilcoxon signed rank test (nonparametric)
    - Mann-Whitney *U* test (nonparametric)
    - Kruskal-Wallis test (nonparametric)

15. **What is a scatterplot?**
    A scatterplot is probably the simplest form of bivariate analysis, but this elementary exercise may convey much meaningful information through the power of the visual medium. A scatterplot can be applied to either continuous or discrete data, or a combination thereof.

16. **What are some other terms for scatterplot?**
    Synonyms for scatterplot include scattergram, scatter diagram, and joint distribution graph.

17. **How is a scatterplot created?**
    To create a scatterplot, simply plot one variable against another on an x-y graph, creating a set of points. This "scatter" of points can then be examined for any visual relationships.
    The power of this method can be illustrated by the scatterplot (Fig. 17-1) of the value of coins in the left pockets of a sample of males in a biostatistics classroom, plotted against their shoe sizes.

18. **How can a scatterplot be useful?**
    A scatterplot can be very useful in the initial analysis of bivariate quantitative data. For example, a quick glance at Figure 17-1 suggests that there is no relationship between the amount of change in the left pocket of a male and his shoe size.

19. **What is a major weakness of the scatterplot?**
    A scatterplot is not quantitative, and it is often useful to have a numeric value indicating the magnitude of relationship or association between the two variables.

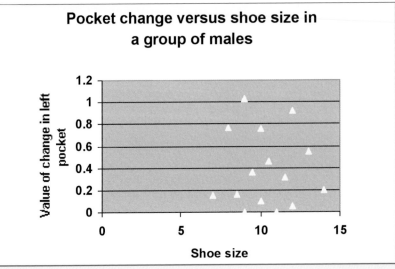

Figure 17-1. Example of scatterplot.

20. **What is the Pearson's correlation coefficient?**
    If we want to examine the relationship or association between two continuous variables in a quantitative fashion, we can calculate the Pearson's correlation coefficient, also known as the product-moment correlation or the population correlation coefficient.

21. **How can we tell which is the dependent (i.e., predictor) variable and which is the dependent (i.e., outcome) variable from a correlation coefficient?**
    We cannot. It is important to note that here we are not making any assumptions about the interdependence of the variables: *neither is considered a function of the other.* In fact, each is considered dependent on the other. We are not so concerned with predicting the value of the variables as we are with determining the association between the two variables.

22. **How is the Pearson's correlation coefficient calculated?**
    Pearson's correlation coefficient can be calculated using one of many available statistics software programs. One formula for its calculation is as follows:

$$r = \frac{\sum(x_i y_i) - \frac{(\sum x_i)(\sum y_i)}{n}}{\left(\sqrt{\sum x_i^2 - \frac{(\sum x_i)^2}{n}}\right)\left(\sqrt{\sum y_i^2 - \frac{(\sum y_i)^2}{n}}\right)}$$

    where r is Pearson's correlation coefficient, and x_i and y_i are the paired values of the associated variables.

23. **What is the range of values for r?**
    The correlation coefficient r must take on a value from -1 to 1. A value of $r = 1$ suggests a perfect positive correlation in which the association between x and y can be described by a straight line with a positive slope. A value of $r = -1$ indicates a perfect negative correlation.

KEY POINTS: PEARSON'S CORRELATION COEFFICIENT

1. Both variables are continuous.

2. Both variables are normally distributed.

3. Data are paired.

24. **What is the purpose of Pearson's correlation coefficient?**

Pearson's correlation coefficient puts into quantitative terms the association implied by a scatterplot of the two variables. A value r = 0 implies no association whatsoever, whereas the values $r = 1$ and $r = -1$ imply perfect positive and negative associations, respectively. Though correlation is valuable in the initial analysis, it is important to note that correlation does not indicate a cause-and-effect relationship, and a correlation of zero does not rule out a relationship between the two variables. Figure 17-2 gives several examples of scatterplots yielding different r values.

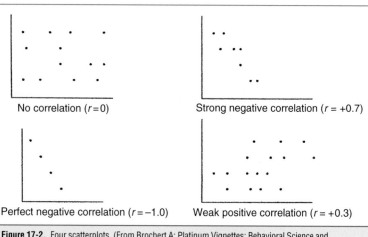

No correlation ($r = 0$) Strong negative correlation ($r = +0.7$)

Perfect negative correlation ($r = -1.0$) Weak positive correlation ($r = +0.3$)

Figure 17-2. Four scatterplots. (From Brochert A: Platinum Vignettes: Behavioral Science and Biostatistics. Philadelphia, Hanley & Belfus, 2003.)

25. **Consider the hypothetic example below, involving paired height and weight data.**

Table 17-1 summarizes the height and weight data for members of a hypothetic biostatistics class. Figure 17-3 depicts the corresponding scatterplot. A positive correlation is implied. For these data,

$$\text{Pearson's } r = \frac{224{,}866 - \frac{(1258) - (3188)}{18}}{\sqrt{88{,}280 - \frac{(1258)^2}{18}} \sqrt{581{,}622 - \frac{(3188)^2}{18}}} = 0.833$$

This value indicates a high (i.e., close to 1) positive correlation or association. Does this imply a cause-and-effect relationship? No. Pearson's correlation makes no assumptions about cause-and-effect or about dependency.

TABLE 17-1. HEIGHT AND WEIGHT DATA FOR MEMBERS OF A HYPOTHETIC BIOSTATISTICS CLASS

Individual	Ht (in), x	Wt (lb), y	x^2	y^2	xy
1	66	152	4356	23,104	10,032
2	72	177	5184	31,329	12,744
3	69	180	4761	32,400	12,420
4	78	224	6084	50,176	17,472
5	68	205	4624	42,025	13,940
6	76	191	5776	36,481	14,516
7	67	174	4489	30,276	11,658
8	74	182	5476	33,124	13,468
9	62	120	3844	14,400	7440
10	60	109	3600	11,881	6540
11	69	172	4761	29,584	11,868
12	67	135	4489	18,225	9045
13	73	198	5329	39,204	14,454
14	69	204	4761	41,616	14,076
15	70	162	4900	26,244	11,340
16	73	211	5329	44,521	15,403
17	71	186	5041	34,596	13,206
18	74	206	5476	42,436	15,244
Σ	1258	3188	88,280	581,622	224,866

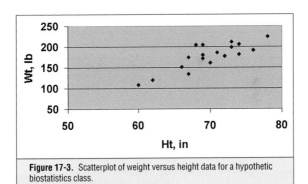

Figure 17-3. Scatterplot of weight versus height data for a hypothetic biostatistics class.

26. You have collected final exam scores and class attendance rates (in percentages) for a group of college students enrolled in an English course. Pearson's correlation for the two variables is 0.23. What is your interpretation? This is a low positive correlation, suggesting little relationship. However, this conclusion is not necessarily true. You should examine the scatterplot to assess more subtle forms of relationship.

27. What is linear regression?

A more sophisticated method for the analysis of two quantitative continuous variables is simple linear regression—"simple" indicating that only two variables are involved. There are some similarities between this method and correlation, but in linear regression one variable is considered dependent on the other.

28. Can linear regression be used as a prediction tool?

In one sense, we are assessing whether the value of the independent variable can be used to predict the value of the dependent variable. An example of an application might be whether or not weight (the independent variable) can be used to predict blood pressure (the dependent variable). In simple linear regression, a "best fit" straight line is determined for the data in which the dependent variable is plotted on the y-axis versus the independent variable on the x-axis. Figure 17-4 shows a "best fit" line drawn for a set of reasonably well-correlated fictitious data.

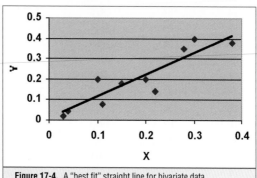

Figure 17-4. A "best fit" straight line for bivariate data, determined by simple linear regression.

29. How is the function of the line in simple linear regression determined?

From algebra, we know that a straight line can be described as $y = mx + b$, where m is the slope and b is the y-intercept. The "best fit" m and b can be determined by a mathematic approach called the method of least squares. This method yields the following values for m and b:

$$m = \frac{\sum(x_i - \bar{x})(y_i - \bar{y})}{\sum(x_i - \bar{x})^2} = \frac{n\sum x_i y_i - (\sum x_i)(\sum y_i)}{n\sum x_i^2 - (\sum x_i)^2}$$

$$b = \bar{y} - m\bar{x}$$

where $\bar{x}$ is the mean of the independent variable and $\bar{y}$ is the mean of the dependent variable. Most regression analysis is performed by use of statistics software.

KEY POINTS: SIMPLE LINEAR REGRESSION

1. Data are continuous and paired.

2. For each x, the associated y values follow a normal distribution.

30. What is the coefficient of determination?

A parameter of significant interest in linear regression is called the coefficient of determination, or r^2. It is a measure of how well the regression equation describes the relationship between the two variables. More specifically, it represents the proportion of variability in the independent variable y (as measured by the difference from the mean) that is accounted for by the regression line. The value of r^2 ranges from 0–1, where 1 indicates that all of the points fall directly on the regression line. Hence, the larger r^2 is, the better the fit of the regression line to the data points. The formula for r^2 is as follows:

$$r^2 = \frac{m^2\left(\sum x_i^2 - \frac{(\sum x_i)^2}{n}\right)}{\sum y_i^2 - \frac{(\sum y_i)^2}{n}}$$

31. **Can statistic testing be used to evaluate the fit of the regression line?**
Statistic testing can also be used to evaluate the fit of the regression line to the data points. This usually takes the form of hypothesis testing—in other words, testing the hypothesis that the slope of the line is zero. If you can reject the null hypothesis that the slope is zero, then a line represents a good or reasonable fit to the data points.

32. **What is the F-test?**
One of the more common test methods for regression line fit employs the F-test. The test statistic is the variance ratio obtained from the ANOVA (analysis of variance) methodology. Most regression analysis today is done by computer, and statistics software usually displays an ANOVA table when linear regression is applied. This table shows the associated p-value for the calculated variance ratio. If this p-value is less than the chosen level of statistic significance (usually designated as the α level and often set at $\alpha = 0.05$), then typically the null hypothesis can be rejected. A t-test can also be applied to test the null hypothesis, but this strategy will not be discussed here.

33. **Give an example problem using the coefficient of determination.**
Let us apply simple regression to the following hypothetic paired, quantitative, continuous data (Table 17-2), consisting of average morning systolic blood pressures, measured the same time, daily, over a period of five days, and body mass index (BMI) for a random sample of males aged 35–45 years not receiving treatment for hypertension. From the data in Table 17-2,

$$m = \frac{(23)[(88,274) - (635)(3146)]}{(23)(18,303) - (635)^2} = 1.837$$

$$b = 136.783 - (1.837)(27.609) = 86.071$$

$$r^2 = \frac{(1.837)^2\left(18,303 - \frac{(635)^2}{23}\right)}{434,852 - \frac{(3146)^2}{23}} = 0.574$$

Thus, the slope and intercept of the linear regression line are given by 1.837 and 86.071, respectively. The coefficient of determination, 0.574, is not close to 1, suggesting that the regression line does not account for a large part of the variation in the independent variable y. The ANOVA table for the data is given below, where df = degrees of freedom, SS = sum of squares, MS = mean square, and VR = variance ratio.

	df	SS	MS	VR	p-Value
Regression	1	2602.811	2602.811	28.305	.0000283
Residual	21	1931.102	91.957		
Total	22	4533.913			

TABLE 17-2.   HYPOTHETIC SYSTOLIC BLOOD PRESSURE VERSUS BMI DATA

Individual No.	BMI (x)	x^2	Systolic BP, mmHg(y)	y^2	xy
1	19	361	118	13,924	2242
2	22	484	122	14,884	2684
3	28	784	128	16,384	3584
4	29	841	134	17,956	3886
5	34	1156	144	20,736	4896
6	32	1024	126	15,876	4032
7	32	1024	162	26,244	5184
8	38	1444	154	23,716	5852
9	22	484	146	21,316	3212
10	21	441	128	16,384	2688
11	18	324	120	14,400	2160
12	35	1225	148	21,904	5180
13	26	676	142	20,164	3692
14	28	784	138	19,044	3864
15	30	900	146	21,316	4380
16	20	400	116	13,456	2320
17	24	576	124	15,376	2976
18	22	484	112	12,544	2464
19	33	1089	154	23,716	5082
20	32	1024	158	24,964	5056
21	25	625	140	19,600	3500
22	28	784	138	19,044	3864
23	37	1369	148	21,904	5476
Σ	635	18,303	3146	434,852	88,274
Average	27.609		136.783		

The details of the ANOVA analytic procedure will not be dealt with here. The above p-value would be statistically significant at $\alpha = 0.05$ (or 0.01, for that matter); thus, the null hypothesis that the slope m is zero can be rejected at these levels of significance. The data points and regression line are shown in Figure 17-5. Interestingly, the p-value is very low, yet the coefficient of determination was not very high (0.574), as you will recall. This is not necessarily a contraindication. The rejection of the null hypothesis only means that if you are going to fit a straight line to the data, the slope of the line would not be zero—it does not necessarily mean that a straight line is the best fit to the data. The relatively low r^2 suggests otherwise.

34. **What is the assumption regarding the values of y (i.e., a dependent variable) for any given value of x (i.e., an independent variable) in linear regression models?**
An important assumption of simple linear regression is that for each value of x, there is a subpopulation of y values that is normally distributed.

KEY POINTS: SPEARMAN'S RANK CORRELATION

1. No assumptions of normality are made for either variable.

2. Variables are continuous or discrete.

3. Data are paired.

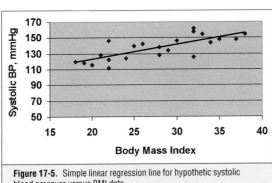

Figure 17-5. Simple linear regression line for hypothetic systolic blood pressure versus BMI data.

35. **How are the nonparametric tests different from the parametric tests discussed (i.e., Pearson's correlation coefficient and linear regression)?**
Nonparametric methods require fewer assumptions, especially with respect to normality (i.e., data following a normal distribution). In addition, nonparametric methods tend to be simple and results can be obtained relatively quickly.

36. **Under what situations are nonparametric tests typically used?**
Typical situations in which nonparametric methods are used include grossly nonnormal data and the analysis of a small sample.

KEY POINTS: WILCOXON SIGNED RANK TEST

1. No assumptions of normality are made about the data (i.e., nonparametric).

2. Data are paired, continuous, or discrete.

3. We want to know whether or not the difference within each pair is significant.

37. **What is Spearman's rank correlation?**
Spearman's rank correlation is a nonparametric analog to Pearson's correlation coefficient. Like Pearson's correlation coefficient, the method attempts to determine if there is an association between two mutually dependent variables, with no assumption that one variable is dependent on another. The variables can be continuous or discrete, and they are paired.

38. **What are the principles underlying Spearman's rank correlation?**
The test is a form of hypothesis testing in which the null hypothesis (H_A) is that there is no rela-tionship between the two variables, and the alternative hypothesis is that there is a relationship. A rank correlation coefficient, r_x, is calculated and used to obtain a test statistic. The test statistic is then compared with a table of critical values to determine the level of statistic significance.

KEY POINTS: MANN-WHITNEY U TEST

1. Data are not assumed to follow a normal distribution.

2. Data are not paired but represent measurements made in two groups that differ in some way (e.g., exposed vs. unexposed).

3. We want to know whether or not the difference in the measurements between the two groups is statistically significant by comparing medians.

---

39. **How is Spearman's rank correlation coefficient calculated?**
The values within each variable are first ranked from 1 to n by magnitude. The difference (d_i) is calculated for each pair of observations (x_i, y_i) by subtracting the rank of y_i from the rank of x_i. Then Spearman's rank correlation coefficient is calculated according to the following formula:

$$r_s = 1 - \frac{6 \sum d_i^2}{n(n^2 - 1)}$$

For $n \le 30$, this becomes the test statistic. For $n > 30$, one must use

$$z = r_s\sqrt{n - 1}$$

40. **Provide an example of calculating Spearman's rank correlation coefficient.**
We can apply Spearman's test to the height and weight data used in a previous example (*see* question 25). For the test, the null hypothesis is that the height and weight are mutually inde-pendent. Our alternative hypothesis is that weight increases with height (i.e., a direct correla-tion). In Table 17-3, each of the values is ranked from lowest to highest within its respective group, beginning with 1. d_i represents the difference between the ranks of x_i and y_i (specifically, $x_i - y_i$). In this example, the method for dealing with ties is also illustrated: one assigns a calcu-lated rank, representing the average of the tied ranks. If the number of ties is not great, the usual formula (in question 39) can be used, as in this case. Since $n \le 30$ for the above data, the test statistic is given by the formula

$$r_s = 1 - \frac{6\,(240.5)}{18\,(18^2 - 1)} = 0.752$$

For $\alpha = 0.05$, the table of Spearman's test statistic critical values gives 0.3994 for $n = 18$. Given the above alternative hypothesis, we are interested in a one-sided test, wherein we will reject the null hypothesis if $r_s > 0.3994$. Because this is true, we reject the null hypothesis and accept the alternative at $p < .05$.

41. **What is Kendall's tau value?**
A method similar to Spearman's rank correlation is Kendall's tau. Like Spearman's rank cor-relation, it is applied to paired data, and the data are assumed to be continuous or discrete.

TABLE 17-3. EXAMPLE OF SPEARMAN'S CORRELATION COEFFICIENT

Individual No.	Ht (in), x	Rank x	Wt (lb), y	Rank y	d	d^2
1	66	3	152	4	−1	2
2	72	12	177	8	4	16
3	69	8	180	9	−1	1
4	78	18	224	18	0	0
5	68	6	205	15	−9	81
6	76	17	191	12	5	25
7	67	4.5	174	7	−2.5	6.25
8	74	15.5	182	10	5.5	30.25
9	62	2	120	2	0	0
10	60	1	109	1	0	0
11	69	8	172	6	2	4
12	67	4.5	135	3	1.5	2.25
13	73	13.5	198	13	0.5	0.25
14	69	8	204	14	−6	36
15	70	10	162	5	5	25
16	73	13.5	211	17	−3.5	12.25
17	71	11	186	11	0	0
18	74	15.5	206	16	−0.5	0.25
Σ						240.5

There are no assumptions of normality. In most cases, the results of Spearman's rank correlation and Kendall's tau are comparable, but the latter is more difficult to calculate.

42. Explain the Wilcoxon signed rank test.
Another nonparametric test for quantitative, paired data is the Wilcoxon signed rank test. In this test, we are trying to assess whether the difference between the values in each pair is significant or not (i.e., the alternative hypothesis is that the difference is not zero). This test is different from both Spearman's rank correlation and Kendall's tau value, both of which involve correlation. However, like Spearman's test, the difference between each pair of data is determined and then ranked. One assigns a positive or negative sign to the ranking, depending on the sign of the original difference. The positive and negative ranks are summed separately and are used to determine the level of statistic significance using a special table.

43. Are there methods to analyze data from two different groups (rather than paired data)?
Yes. Up to now we have focused on nonparametric methods of analysis of paired data. Now consider the Mann-Whitney U test, a nonparametric test that is used to determine whether two sets of continuous or discrete data are significantly "different." An example of an application of the Mann-Whitney U test would be the measurement of a characteristic (e.g., weight) in exposed and unexposed groups. As noted above, the variable being measured or collected is quantitative and either continuous or discrete. The two sets of data are assumed to be independent and randomly drawn. The statistics of interest in this test are the *medians* of both sets of data, and the test determines whether or not the difference in the medians is statistically significant at a given level.

44. **Is there a nonparametric test for comparing the medians of more than two samples?**
Yes. The Kruskal-Wallis test is another nonparametric test that can be used to determine whether the medians from two samples are different. Unlike the Mann-Whitney U test, it is not limited to just two samples. However, as with the Mann-Whitney U test, the samples are assumed to be random, independent samples.

45. **Is it possible to analyze two groups of categoric data?**
Yes. Often statistic analysis is performed on data involving two categoric variables. An example is the absence or presence of a cough in cases of group A beta-hemolytic streptococcal pharyngitis versus nongroup A beta-hemolytic streptococcal pharyngitis. This type of data naturally leads to representation in tables (called contingency tables) in which the categories are represented as rows and columns. For example, the above example would be depicted in the following 2 × 2 contingency table:

	+ Cough	− Cough
Group A streptococcal pharyngitis	A	B
Nongroup A streptococcal pharyngitis	C	D

46. **Explain the above contingency table.**
A–D represent the count of cases, with the pair of characteristics determined by the intersection of the rows and columns. For instance, A subjects had both a cough and group A streptococcal pharyngitis, whereas C subjects had both a cough and nongroup A streptococcal pharyngitis. The total subjects with cough is A + C, and the total number of subjects in the study is A + B + C + D.

47. **What is the chi-square statistic?**
The chi-square statistic is a nonparametric test of bivariate count or frequency data. This method of modeling examines the disparity between the actual count frequencies and the expected count frequencies when the null hypothesis of no difference between the groups is true. We can apply the chi-square test to determine whether an association exists between group A beta-hemolytic streptococcal pharyngitis and coughing.

48. **How is the chi-square statistic calculated?**
In this method, a chi-square test statistic is calculated by the following formula:

$$\chi^2 = \sum_{i=1}^{r} \sum_{j=1}^{c} \frac{(O_{ij} - E_{ij})^2}{E_{ij}}$$

where $E_{ij} = \frac{O_{i.} \times O_{.j}}{n}$, r = number of rows, c = number of columns, O_{ij} = the observed number for the intersection of the ith row and the jth column, E_{ij} = expected number for the intersection of the ith row and the jth column, $O_{i.}$ = sum of terms for the ith row (in the table above, O_1 = sum of the first row of entries = A + B), $O_{.j}$ = sum of the jth *column* entries (in the table above, $O_{.2}$ = sum of entries in the second column = B + D), and n = the total number of cases (above, n = A + B + C + D).

49. **How is the calculated chi-square statistic used?**
Once the chi-square statistic is calculated, the probability that the frequency counts in the table are due to chance (i.e., that the null hypothesis is true) can be determined for the number of degrees of freedom from a standard chi-square table. For any given number of degrees of freedom, the higher the chi-square statistic, the more unlikely the frequency disparities are due to chance.

KEY POINTS: CHI-SQUARE TEST

1. Variables are categoric.

2. Data represent counts and can be represented in a table of r rows and c columns, an $r \times c$ contingency table.

3. Cochran's criteria should be met to apply the basic chi-square test.

50. **What are Cochran's criteria?**
Cochran's criteria should be fulfilled if the chi-square test statistic is to be used as noted above. These criteria are
- All expected values in each cell have a frequency count ≥1.
- 80% of expected values in each cell should be ≥5.
    The number of terms or cells for summation will be given by $r \times c$ in general. For the above table, therefore, there would be 2×2, or 4, terms for summation for the chi-square statistic.

51. **What is the maximum number of rows or columns for which a chi-square statistic can be calculated?**
There is no theoretic limit to the number of rows or columns (a variable could easily have more than two categories), and the computation can become tedious. Statistics software is highly recommended.

52. **Is there a simplified formula for calculating the chi-square statistic in the 2×2 contingency table?**
Thankfully, yes. For the above 2×2 table, the formula simplifies to

$$\chi^2 = \frac{n(ad - bc)^2}{(a + c)(b + d)(a + b)(c + d)}$$

53. **How can one determine the degrees of freedom in any contingency table?**
To apply the chi-square test, one must determine the degrees of freedom, given by the formula $df = (r-1)(c-1)$. For a 2×2 table, $df = 1$; for a 3×3 table there are $(3 - 1)(3 - 1) = 4$ degrees of freedom. After choosing the level of significance (α), one should consult the chi-square distribution to determine whether the null hypothesis of no association can be rejected.

54. **Provide an example problem using the chi-square statistic in a 2×2 table.**
Hypothesis: Vitamin C supplements reduce a person's susceptibility to the common cold. Consider 90 subjects selected at random and grouped on the basis of whether or not they take vitamin C supplements. A 2×2 table for this sample is given below:

	+Common Cold	−Common Cold
+**Vitamin C supplements**	12	23
+**Vitamin C supplements**	28	27

The chi-square statistic is calculated using the equation in question 52:

$$\chi^2 = \frac{n(ad - bc)^2}{(a + c)(b + d)(a + b)(c + d)} = \frac{90\,[(12)(27) - (23)(28)]^2}{(40)(50)(35)(55)}$$

$$\chi^2 = \frac{9,216,000}{3,850,000}$$

$$\chi^2 = 2.39$$

Chi-square = 2.39, with $(2 - 1)(2 - 1) = 1$ degree of freedom.

Now, checking Appendix C for chi-square distributions and assuming that $p = .05$ (i.e., a 95% confidence level that the difference is not due to chance), we find that the chi-square statistic must be at least 3.841 to show a significant difference. Therefore, we must accept the null hypothesis that vitamin C has no effect on the susceptibility to the common cold.

55. What is the Yates correction?

The Yates correction is a correction for continuity for 2×2 tables. Some experts believe that this correction is necessary, especially when frequency counts are low, because the chi-square statistic is a discrete value (since it is calculated from integer data) whose distribution is being approximated by a continuous distribution (i.e., the chi-square distribution). Mathematically, the Yates correction is simply accomplished by subtracting 0.5 from the absolute value of the difference between the observed (O) and expected (E) values before squaring the denominator.

$$\text{Yates } \chi^2 = \sum \frac{(|\,O - E\,| - .5)^2}{E}$$

56. Should I always use the Yates correction for continuity when performing chi-square tests?

It is up to you. Belief that this correction is necessary is not universal. In fact, for large counts in contingency tables, it is probably not required, although it is typically suggested when smaller counts are analyzed.

57. What if Cochran's criteria are not met?

If Cochran's criteria for using the chi-square technique are not met (e.g., if the counts in some cells are too low), one can apply the Fisher exact test for 2×2 tables.

58. What about cases in which we are analyzing categoric data that are, in fact, paired?

As noted above, the chi-square test does not assume paired or matched data. In the case of paired or matched categoric data, the McNemar test can be applied. In this case, a particular characteristic or quality is assessed in the same individual under different conditions, or in individuals who have been matched for potential confounding factors.

59. How about an example of the proper use of the McNemar test?

One example is a study of the occurrence of headaches in matched individuals after the ingestion of the same medication. Another might be the occurrence of ear infections (*otitis media*) in individuals at the ages of 5 and 15 years.

	+Ear infections at age 15	−Ear infections at age 15
+Ear infections at age 5	A	B
+Ear infections at age 5	C	D

Using the McNemar test, one would assess whether there is a statistically significant difference in the occurrence of ear infections at the two ages in the sample. If the sample is large, the McNemar test statistic would be calculated as follows:

$$\chi^2 = \frac{(b - c)^2}{b + c}$$

After selecting the level of statistic significance (usually $\alpha = 0.05$), the chi-square distribution would be used to determine whether the null hypothesis of no difference can be rejected.

60. **Can the McNemar test be used if there is more than one possible outcome?**
Although our examples involved variables with two outcomes, the McNemar test has been extended to variables with more than two outcomes.

61. **Describe logistic regression.**
Logistic regression is a statistical method analogous to linear regression for the analysis of categorical data. In logistic regression, the dependent variable is categorical (in the simplest case, dichotomous, or having two outcomes like absence or presence of disease). The independent variables can be categorical, or else continuous or discrete. Like linear regression, logistic regression is a powerful tool that has been widely used in medical research. Independent variables can be assessed for their contribution to the outcome of the dependent variable (e.g., the presence of disease).

62. **Can logistic regression be performed when more than one independent variable may potentially affect the outcome?**
Yes. In the simplest case, logistic regression involves the modeling of a dichotomous dependent variable on a single independent variable that is categoric or quantitative. In most applications, multiple independent variables are assessed in the regression model.

63. **Can logistic regression models be used to quantify risk?**
Another important and very useful feature of logistic regression is the ability to calculate odds ratios of an outcome of the dependent variable (e.g., lung cancer) given specified values of one of the independent variables (e.g., smoking vs. nonsmoking) while controlling for the values of the other independent variables (e.g., alcohol intake, family history, and antioxidant use).

WEBSITES

1. http://www.mste.uiuc.edu/hill/dstat/dstat.html

2. http://www.davidmlane.com/hyperstat/index.html

3. http://www.emedicine.com/emerg/topic758.htm

BIBLIOGRAPHY

1. Brochert A: Platinum Vignettes: Behavioral Science and Biostatistics. Philadelphia, Hanley & Belfus, 2003.
2. Daly LE, Bourke GJ: Interpretation and Uses of Medical Statistics, 5th ed. Oxford, Blackwell Science Ltd., 2000.
3. Kirkwood BR: Essentials of Medical Statistics. Oxford, Blackwell Science Ltd., 1988.
4. Norman GR, Streiner DL: Biostatistics: The Bare Essentials, 2nd ed. Toronto, B.C. Decker, 2000.

CHAPTER 18

MULTIVARIABLE AND MULTIVARIATE ANALYSIS

Robbie Ali, MD, MPH, MPPM

1. **What is multivariable analysis?**
   According to Katz, "Multivariable analysis is a tool for determining the relative contributions of different causes to a single event or outcome."

   Katz MH: Multivariable Analysis: A Practical Guide for Clinicians. Cambridge, Cambridge University Press, 1999.

2. **What is the difference between multivariable and multivariate analysis?**
   Multivariable analysis is used for data with one dependent outcome variable but more than one independent variable. *Multivariate* analysis is used for data with more than one dependent outcome variable as well as more than one independent variable.

3. **List the common uses of multivariable analysis.**
   - To quantify associations: indicates how well several independent variables, separately and together, explain or predict the variation in one dependent variable (e.g., goodness of fit of a model).
   - To look for interaction between independent variables: interaction occurs when two or more independent variables, when present together, produce an effect different from a simple addition of their individual effects.
   - To adjust for potential confounders in a controlled study: a *confounder* is a factor (e.g., alcohol intake) that leads to an observed correlation between two variables (e.g., smoking and cirrhosis) that does not stem from a causal relation between them, but rather from their common relation to the confounder.
   - To develop models to predict values or probabilities of certain outcomes: for example, multivariable analysis might allow prediction of how likely it is that a cancer patient who has a certain set of characteristics and who receives a certain treatment might recover.

KEY POINTS: USES OF MULTIVARIABLE ANALYSIS

1. To quantify associations.

2. To look for interaction between independent variables.

3. To adjust for potential confounders in a controlled study.

4. To develop models to predict values or probabilities of certain outcomes.

4. **How can I decide what type of multivariable analysis to use?**
   Look at your data! Figure 18-1 summarizes the following guidelines:
   - If the dependent variable consists of dichotomous categoric data (two outcomes, e.g., yes or no, diseased or well, or live or die), you can use logistic regression.
   - If the dependent variable also includes a time factor (e.g., a survival curve), you can use the Cox proportional hazards model.

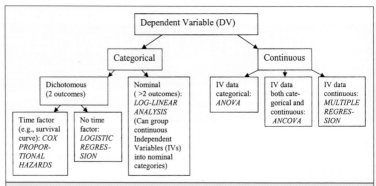

Figure 18-1. How to choose the appropriate type of multivariable analysis. (Adapted from Jekel JF, Katz DL, Elmore JG: Epidemiology, Biostatistics, and Preventive Medicine. Philadelphia, W.B. Saunders, 2001, pp 209–217.)

- If the dependent variable consists of nominal categoric data (i.e., more than two outcomes), you can use log-linear analysis. If some or all of the independent variables are continuous, you may have to group them into nominal categories to do so.
- If both the dependent and independent variables consist of continuous data, use multiple regression.
- For a continuous dependent variable with categoric independent variables, use analysis of variance (ANOVA), or if there are both categoric and continuous independent variables, use analysis of covariance (ANCOVA).

5. **What is the name given to a line describing the relationship between a dependent continuous variable and an independent variable, which allows the prediction of the dependent variable from the independent one?**
   A regression line.

6. **Give a simple equation for a regression line and explain its elements.**

   $$Y = a + bX + E$$

   where Y is the dependent variable, a is a constant equal to the y-intercept (i.e., value of Y when X = 0), b is the line's slope (i.e., regression coefficient), X is the independent variable, and E is the error term.

7. **Are regression lines always straight lines?**
   No. The above equation describes a straight line. Other regression equations describe curves; for example,
   - Parabolas: $Y = a + bX + cX^2$
   - Exponential curves: $Log(Y) = a + bX$
   - Logarithmic curves: $Y = a + b\,Log(X)$
   - Geometric curves: $Log(Y) = a + b\,Log(X)$

   Such regression equations are used to *model data* of relationships between dependent and independent variables as equations of approximating curves.

8. **List three data requirements for regression analysis.**
   1. The dependent variable must be continuous.
   2. The dependent variable must be normally distributed (unless advanced techniques are used).

KEY POINTS: DATA AND TESTS

1. If the dependent variable consists of dichotomous categoric data, you can use logistic regression.

2. If the dependent variable also includes a time factor (e.g., a survival curve), you can use the Cox proportional hazards model.

3. If the dependent variable consists of nominal categoric data (i.e., more than two outcomes), you can use log-linear analysis. If some or all of the independent variables are continuous, you may have to group them into nominal categories to do this.

4. If both the dependent and independent variables consist of continuous data, use multiple regression.

5. For a continuous dependent variable with categoric independent variables, use ANOVA (or ANCOVA, if there are both categoric and continuous independent variables).

    3. The variability of the dependent variable should stay the same for all values of the independent variable (unless advanced techniques are used).

9. **How are the data requirements for regression different from those of correlation?**
For correlation, both the dependent variable and the independent variable must be normally distributed. For regression analysis, only the dependent variable need be normally distributed. The independent variable does not need to be normally distributed; in fact, the researcher can select its value.

10. **What is the term given to a measure of a particular regression model's goodness of fit, equal to the proportion of the variation in the dependent variable (i.e., explained variation/total variation, ranging from 0–1) that the model explains?**
Coefficient of determination (R^2). For example, in study 1 with sample population 1, a scatterplot of outcome Y (child's height) versus factor X1 (child's age) may show points that cluster around a line, with an R^2 near to 1, whereas in study 2 with sample population 2, a scatterplot of outcome Y2 (intelligence quotient) versus factor X2 (blood pressure) may show a cloud of points with no real relationship to a line, with an R^2 near to 0.

11. **What is the name given to the type of analysis that describes a relationship between a dependent continuous variable and *two or more* independent variables, which allows the prediction of the dependent variable from the independent ones?**
Multiple regression.

12. **Give a simple example of a multiple regression equation and explain its elements.**

$$Y = a + b1X1 + b2X2 + b3\,X3$$

where Y is the dependent variable (e.g., blood pressure); *a* is a constant; X1, X2, and X3 are independent variables (e.g., age, race, and gender); and *b1, b2,* and *b3* are regression coefficients that serve as weighting factors for the relative contributions of X1, X2, and X3 to outcome Y.

KEY POINTS: SIMPLE REGRESSION

1. A simple regression line describes the relationship between a dependent continuous variable and an independent variable.

2. An example of a simple equation for a regression line is Y = $a + b$X, where Y is the dependent variable, a is a constant (i.e., the y-intercept), b is the line's slope (i.e., regression coefficient), and X is the independent variable.

3. For regression analysis, the dependent variable must be continuous. For a unit change in X, there will be a b unit change in Y.

4. Unless special techniques are used, the dependent variable must also be normally distributed and have variability that stays the same for all values of the independent variable.

5. The coefficient of determination (R^2) describes a regression model's goodness of fit as the proportion of the variation in the dependent variable (i.e., explained variation/total variation, ranging from 0–1) that the model explains. The closer R^2 is to 1, the better the model explains the variation.

13. **How are regression coefficients (b) estimated in multiple regression equations?**
By the *ordinary least squares* method: minimizing the sum of squared residuals (i.e., error terms) between the regression plane (analogous to regression line) and observed values for each dependent variable. This gives the equation that "best fits" the observed data.

14. **In a multiple regression equation, what does it mean if the *p*-value for the regression coefficients of one or more independent variables is small (i.e., < .05)?**
It means that there is sufficient evidence in the data to show that the independent variable has an association with the dependent variable that is greater than what would be expected by chance alone; thus, we reject the null hypothesis.

15. **Why is this concept important in model building with multiple regression equations?**
In model building, we can progressively add independent variables to a regression equation and keep or reject them based on whether or not their regression coefficients are statistically significant.

16. **To analyze how several independent variables predict a *dichotomous* dependent (i.e., outcome) variable, what is the statistic method of choice?**
Logistic regression.

17. **What is logistic regression?**
Logistic regression is a tool used to find the best-fitting model for a relationship between one or more independent variables and *a dependent variable that is dichotomous, or binary*. A dichotomous dependent variable has only two possible outcomes (e.g., yes or no, true or false, success or failure, or live or die). The dependent variable in logistic regression is also called a *dummy* variable, which means it can be coded as either 0 or 1.

KEY POINTS: MULTIPLE LINEAR REGRESSION

1. Multiple linear regression describes a relationship between a dependent continuous variable and two or more independent variables, which allows the prediction of the dependent variable from the independent ones.

2. A simple example of a multiple regression equation is $Y = a + b1X1 + b2X2 + b3X3$, where Y is the dependent variable; a is a constant; $b1$, $b2$, and $b3$ are regression coefficients; and X1, X2, and X3 are independent variables. For a unit change in X1, there will be a b unit change in Y (holding X2 and X3 constant).

3. Regression coefficients (b) are estimated in multiple regression equations by the *ordinary least squares* method.

4. In building models, unless there is significant interaction between independent variables, an independent variable with a regression coefficient not significantly different from 0 ($p > .05$) can be removed. If $p < .05$, then the variable should be retained.

18. **How is the logistic regression equation different from the linear regression equation?**
    The logistic regression equation is a nonlinear transformation of the linear regression equation. This logit transformation results in a "logit" regression model instead of the "probit" regression model of a standard normal distribution. Graphically, the logit transformation converts the straight-line model of linear regression into an S-shaped logistic model, asymptotic to the Y values of 0 and 1 (Fig. 18-2).

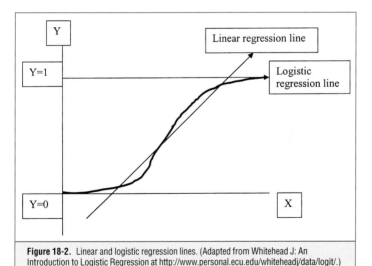

Figure 18-2. Linear and logistic regression lines. (Adapted from Whitehead J: An Introduction to Logistic Regression at http://www.personal.ecu.edu/whiteheadj/data/logit/.)

19. **Give an example of how a linear regression equation can be transformed into a logistic regression equation.**
    Consider the following linear regression equation:

Y (dichotomous dependent variable) = a (constant) + $b1$X1 + $b2$X2 +... + E (error)

It can be transformed into a logistic regression equation so that, if p is the probability of the Y outcome occurring (Y = 1),

Log odds ratio = Logit (p) = ln[$p/(1 − p)$] = $a + b1$X1 + $b2$X2 + ...+ E (error)

and, taking the exponential of both sides,

Odds = [$p/(1 − p)$] = exp$a$ exp$b1$X1 exp$b2$expX2...exp$e$

where the elements of the equation have the following meaning:

- X1, X2,. . . are the independent variables
- $b1$, $b2$,, are the regression coefficients of the independent variables
- ln is the natural logarithm (i.e., the log of exp)
- exp = 2.71828. . . .

20. **Remind me what natural log (ln) and exp = 2.71828... are all about. Why are they used in logistic regression?**

Exp (i.e., exponential, sometimes also called e) is the base of the natural log system. The numeric value of exp is equal to an added series of inverse factorials: $1 + 1/1 + 1/(1 \times 2) + 1/(1 \times 2 \times 3) +...+ 1/(1 \times 2 \times 3 \times...\times \infty)$, with ∞ = infinity. Exp has a unique property among numbers because exp$x$ (i.e., the log function with base e) is the only log function which is *equal to its own derivative*. This means that the slope of a line tangent to exp$x$ (i.e., the rate of change of exp$x$) at any value of x is equal to exp$x$. It also means that the natural log of e^X is x; thus, the natural log of $e(e^1) = 1$ and the natural log of $1(e^0) = 0$.

When something changes at a rate the same as its own value, it is said to be undergoing exponential growth (such as occurs in continuous compounding of interest) or exponential decay (such as occurs with radioactive materials). Natural logs are useful in modeling functions such as these and for looking at their slopes through differential equations. The b regression coefficient in logistic regression is such a slope. Logistic transformation of linear regression lines with natural logs corrects several problems that arise with linear regression (*see* question 21).

A more in-depth, but still quite readable, account of natural logs can be found in *e: The Story of a Number* by Eli Maor (Princeton, 1998). It is compelling material, but it will not be on the boards!

21. **List three reasons why logistic regression and the logit model are better than linear regression and ordinary least squares for predicting probabilities with a dichotomous dependent variable.**

1. In the linear model, error is *not* normally distributed. Not good for regression! The logit transformation takes care of this.
2. In the linear model, the error terms are *heteroskedastic* (i.e., variance of the dependent variable changes with different values of the independent variables). Not good for regression, either! The logit transformation takes care of this, too.
3. In the linear model, predicted probabilities can be *greater than 1 or less than 0*, a theoretic impossibility. After logit transformation, estimated probabilities will be between 0 and 1.

22. **How can a logit coefficient (e.g., exp b) be interpreted?**

As an odds ratio (OR), Exp$b$ (i.e., 2.71828... to the b power) is the OR of the individual coefficient b for the independent variable X. It tells the *relative* amount by which the overall odds ratio, or the probability that Y = 1/(probability that Y = 0), changes when the value of the independent variable X is increased by 1 unit, with all other factors remaining unchanged. Note that in logistic regression, the b coefficients represent *maximum likelihood*, and not ordinary least squares, as in linear regression.

KEY POINTS: LOGISTIC REGRESSION

1. Logistic regression is typically used to find the best-fitting model for a relationship between one or more independent variables and a dependent variable that is dichotomous, or binary.

2. The logistic regression equation is a nonlinear transformation of the linear regression equation. This "logit" transformation results in a "logit" regression model instead of the "probit" regression model of a standard-normal distribution.

3. A logit coefficient (e.g., exp$b$) can be interpreted as an odds ratio that tells the *relative* amount by which the overall odds ratio changes when the value of the independent variable X is increased by 1 unit.

4. The statistic significance of the b coefficient can be tested using the Wald statistic; in other words, $[b/\text{standard error}_b]^2$.

5. In building models, as in linear regression, unless there is significant interaction between independent variables, an independent variable with a regression coefficient not significantly different from 0 (i.e., $p > .05$) can be removed. If $p < .05$, then the variable should be retained.

23. **How is the statistic significance of the b coefficient tested in logistic regression?**

By using the Wald statistic: $[b/\text{standard error}_b]^2$. In modeling, an independent variable with a regression coefficient not significantly different from 0 (i.e., $p > .05$) can be removed from the regression model. If $p < .05$, the variable contributes significantly to the prediction of the outcome variable and should be retained.

24. **When is analysis of variance (ANOVA) used? How does it work?**

ANOVA is used with data when the dependent variable is continuous (e.g., blood pressure) and all independent variables are categoric (e.g., different types of medication). ANOVA can test for significant differences among means in several groups without increasing the type I error rate (as would result from conducting multiple t-tests). One-way ANOVA is used when there is one categoric independent variable, whereas N-way ANOVA is used when there is more than one.

ANOVA describes the total variation in study data by *partitioning* it into variation explained by the independent variables (i.e., group differences), variation caused by interaction between independent variables, and variation caused by random error (i.e., chance). The component variations are then compared to the variation caused by the random error by means of the F statistic.

25. **What multivariable methods use the F statistic?**

ANOVA and analysis of covariance (ANCOVA). The F-ratio is equal to between-groups variance divided by within-groups variance. Variance for each of these is simply the sum of squares (SS) divided by the degrees of freedom (df):

$$F\text{-ratio} = \frac{SS/df \text{ (between-groups)}}{SS/df \text{ (within-groups)}}$$

The F-test, like the Student's t-test, compares means, but it can compare more than two means at the same time. It tests whether the variation between group means is due to chance alone or to actual differences between the groups. The p-values for the F statistic can be looked up in an F-table.

26. **How many degrees of freedom does the *F* statistic have?**
Two. One for between-group variance and one for within-group variance.

27. **What does it mean if the *F*-ratio is much greater than 1?**
It means that the null hypothesis that there are no significant differences between groups should be rejected. Conversely, if the *F*-statistic is close to 1, the null hypothesis cannot be rejected, either because the study was too small or because the study variance was completely explainable by chance and not by real differences in groupings using the independent variables.

28. **When is analysis of covariance used? How does it work?**
ANCOVA is used when the data to be analyzed consist of a continuous dependent variable along with *both* categoric and continuous independent variables. The method first adjusts for the continuous independent variable or variables (e.g., age or weight) through regression and then analyzes the variance for the categoric variables as in ANOVA, using the *F*-test to compare between-group and within-group variance.

KEY POINTS: ANALYSIS OF VARIANCE (ANOVA)

1. ANOVA is used with data for which the dependent variable is continuous and all independent variables are categoric.

2. ANOVA uses the *F* statistic.

3. The *F* statistic has two degrees of freedom, one for between-group variance and one for within-group variance.

4. Reject the null hypothesis if the *F*-ratio is much greater than 1.

29. **What statistic method is often used to analyze covariates in survival curves (e.g., Kaplan-Meier)?**
The *Cox proportional hazards model*, which is a form of multivariable regression model used to analyze survival curves and clinic trials with a dichotomous outcome (e.g., dead vs. alive or diseased vs. disease-free). It allows comparison of subjects with differing characteristics and different starting and ending points of observation over time.

30. **What is a hazard function?**
In a study that looks at subjects' survival times (or disease-free periods), a hazard function is a way of estimating survival (or the disease-free period) for each subject. This hazard function is an exponential function. For a given subject, its value depends on the value of the baseline hazard and on the values of the regression coefficients (i.e., expβ) of that subject's independent variables (i.e., covariates).

31. **What assumptions does the Cox proportional hazards model make?**
The model assumes that each subject's survival (or disease-free period) can be estimated by a hazard function. The model also assumes *proportionality of hazards*, hence the name. This means that it assumes there is a baseline or underlying hazard rate (e.g., risk of death per year of observation) with a multiplicative relationship to some function of the covariates for each subject. This also means that the value of each covariate represents a relative risk that is *constant over time*, and that two individuals with particular values for the covariates will have a ratio of the estimated hazards that is constant over time.

32. **What key assumptions does the Cox proportional hazards model *not* make?**
The model makes no assumptions about the nature or shape of the hazard function or survival distribution. It also makes no assumption that subjects are under observation for the same lengths of time or that subjects are similar to one another; rather, it controls for these subject differences (by treating them as independent variables) and for different periods of observation.

KEY POINTS: OTHER METHODS

1. Analysis of covariance (ANCOVA) is used when the data to be analyzed consist of a continuous dependent variable along with *both* categoric and continuous independent variables.

2. The Cox proportional hazards model is a form of multivariable regression model used to analyze survival curves (e.g., Kaplan-Meier), for example, and clinical trials with a dichotomous outcome over time (e.g., dead vs. alive or diseased vs. disease-free).

3. Log-linear analysis is helpful in analyzing factors in frequency tables (i.e., cross-tabulations) in terms of interactions, statistic significance, and model-fitting.

4. Discriminant function analysis is used to detect which of several variables best discriminate between two or more groups.

5. Cluster analysis is used to organize variables into relatively homogeneous groups, or "clusters."

6. Canonical correlation is used to explore the relationship between two *sets* of variables.

33. **In reality, are the hazard rates associated with subject characteristics (i.e., covariates) always constant over time?**
Not necessarily. In a given study, the risks associated with some covariates may be *time-dependent*. For example, in a 10-year prospective study of outdoor air pollution and the development of asthma in children, parental smoking as a covariate may represent a greater risk to younger children. Unless one accounts for such changes in risk over time, the validity of the analysis may be called into question.

34. **What statistic method is helpful in analyzing factors in frequency tables (i.e., cross-tabulations) in terms of interactions, statistic significance, and model-fitting?**
Log-linear analysis. A multiway frequency table (i.e., a cross-tabulation table of two or more factors) is one way to summarize data about interacting variables (e.g., in a study of meningitis patients, frequencies of presenting symptoms such as fever, headache, and neck pain according to patient age, race, and gender). In log-linear modeling, a multiway frequency table and its observed values are "translated" through *logarithmic* transformations into several main effects and interaction effects that add together *linearly* to form *log-linear* equations. These derived log-linear equations thus express relationships between factors in the frequency table in terms very similar to those used in ANOVA and allow testing for statistically significant relationships.

35. **What statistic tool helps tell which of several variables *best discriminates* between two or more naturally occurring groups?**
Discriminant function analysis, which is a multivariate technique used to detect which of several variables best discriminates between two or more groups. For example, a researcher may want

to detect which variables (e.g., age, gender, or race) in the backgrounds of patients with a certain disease best discriminate between those who (1) recover completely, (2) go into remission, or (3) do poorly. Discriminant function analysis is computationally similar to multivariate analysis of variance (MANOVA).

36. **What statistic tool involves taxonomies, similarity matrices, and dendrograms?**
    Cluster analysis, which is a multivariate tool used to organize variables into relatively homogeneous groups, or "clusters." It involves the generation of a *similarity matrix.* A cluster analysis produces a *dendrogram* (i.e., tree diagram). The clusters formed represent groups with members more similar to one another than to members of other clusters.

37. **What statistic tool is used to compare two *sets* of variables?**
    Canonical correlation, which is a multivariate tool used to explore the relationship between two *sets* of variables. An example might be the relationship between (1) a list of various risk factors for asthma (e.g., pollens, air pollution, cold, and exercise) and (2) a list of developed symptoms of asthma (e.g., wheeze, cough, and dyspnea). Canonical correlation involves the computation of *eigenvalues,* which tell how much variance is accounted for by the correlation between the several variates in the two lists.

ACKNOWLEDGMENT

The author wishes to thank Abdus Wahed, PhD, Department of Biostatistics, Graduate School of Public Health, University of Pittsburgh, for his helpful suggestions and comments on this chapter.

WEBSITES

1. http://www.statsoft.com/textbook/stathome.html

2. http://personal.ecu.edu/whiteheadj/data/logit/

BIBLIOGRAPHY

1. Jekel JF, Katz DL, Elmore JG: Epidemiology, Biostatistics, and Preventive Medicine. Philadelphia, W.B. Saunders, 2001, pp 209–217.
2. Katz MH: Multivariable Analysis: A Practical Guide for Clinicians. Cambridge, Cambridge University Press, 1999.

CHAPTER 19

SURVIVAL ANALYSIS

Ashita Tolwani, MD, MSc

1. **What is survival analysis?**

   Survival analysis is a statistical method for studying the time between entry to a study and a subsequent event. The variable of interest is time until an event occurs. The event is typically referred to as a failure. A common example is time from treatment to death.

2. **What is one characteristic of survival analysis that makes it unique?**

   Survival analysis must deal with the unequal observation time of the subjects under study. This fact makes survival analysis incompatible with many conventional study designs.

3. **Is survival analysis used only in mortality studies?**

   No. Other examples include
   - Time from treatment of a disease to relapse
   - Length of unemployment, measured from date of layoff
   - Time to failure of a piece of equipment

4. **What are other terms for survival data?**
   - Time-to-event data
   - Lifetime data
   - Failure time data
   - Reliability data
   - Duration data
   - Event history data

5. **What are some of the goals of survival analysis?**
   - Making predictions about a population
   - Comparing the effect of treatment between two groups
   - Investigating the importance of specific characteristics on survival

6. **Why cannot standard regression techniques be used to determine whether certain variables are correlated with survival or failure times?**
   - The dependent variable of interest (i.e., survival or failure time) is not normally distributed; survival times usually follow an exponential, Weibull, or Gompertz distribution.
   - Standard regression techniques fail to take censoring into account and can produce bias in estimates of the distributions of survival time and related quantities.

7. **What is meant by censored data?**

   In an experiment in which subjects are followed over time until an event of interest occurs, it is not always possible to follow every subject until the event is observed. If a subject is no longer followed, for any reason, all that is known is that the time to the event was at least as long as the time to when the subject was last observed. The observed time to the event under such circumstances is unknown and thus *censored*.

8. **Can we ignore the censored data when performing the analysis?**
No. These observations cannot be ignored as they carry important information despite their incompleteness. For each subject, we at least know that the subject's time to event is greater than time on observation.

9. **What are the essential data required to perform a survival analysis?**
   - Time of study entry
   - Study endpoint
   - Date of last follow-up
   - Patient status as of the time of last follow-up (i.e., censored or uncensored)

10. **Give three reasons why censoring might occur.**
    - A subject does not experience the event before the study ends.
    - A person is lost to follow-up during the study period.
    - A person withdraws from the study.

11. **What is the main assumption of censoring?**
We assume the time of censoring and time of failure are independent. In other words, subjects who are censored are assumed to have the same underlying survival curve after their censoring time as patients who are not censored; they are at the same risk of failure as those who stay in the study. This is known as noninformative censoring.

12. **What is the difference between right censoring, left censoring, and interval censoring?**
    - *Right censoring* occurs when the observation stops before the event is observed. At time t, right censoring means true survival time is at least t.
    - *Left censoring* occurs when the observation does not begin until after the event has occurred. Left censored at time t means that the true survival time is at most t. For example, a study involving patients infected with hepatitis C may start follow-up when the subject first tests positive for the hepatitis C virus, but the exact time of first exposure to the virus is unknown. Thus, the survival time is censored on the left side.
    - *Interval censoring* means true survival is known only to have occurred somewhere within a known interval of time.

13. **What is the most common type of censuring?**
Right censoring is the most common type of censoring.

14. **In Figure 19-1, letters A–E represent patients in a survival study. Which patients are censored?**
    - Patients B and E reach "failure." Patient B is observed from the start of the study. Patient E enters the study at year 3 and is followed until reaching "failure" at year 5.5. There is no censoring.
    - Patient D enters the study at year 2 and is followed until year 4, when he is lost to follow-up; his censored time is 2 years.
    - Patients A and C are followed to the end of the study. For patient A, the survival time is censored because it is at least 7 years. Patient C enters the study at year 2 and is followed for the remainder of the study without reaching "failure;" his censored time is 5 years.
    In summary, patients B and E reach failure, and patients A, C, and D are censored.

15. **What are the types of right censoring?**
    - *Simple type I* censoring occurs when all individuals are censored at the same fixed time. It usually occurs when a population is followed during some fixed time interval.

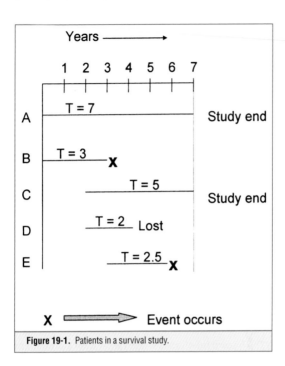

Figure 19-1. Patients in a survival study.

- *Progressive type I* censoring occurs when individuals enter at different times and are followed until some fixed date. The outcome of interest is the duration between entry and event.
- *Type II* censoring occurs when a study ends when there are a prespecified number of events.
- *Random censoring* occurs when the study is designed to end after a fixed time, but censored subjects do not all have the same censoring time. The time of censoring and the survival time T are independent.

16. **How can censoring bias the results?**
As the number of censored patients in a study increases, any differences between the censored and uncensored patients may increase the chance of bias. Conventionally, the number of patients censored should be less than 5% of the total.

17. **What is a survival function?**
A survival function describes the proportion of subjects surviving to or beyond a given time.

18. **How do you mathematically define the survival function?**
The survival function is defined by $S(t) = P(T > t)$, the probability that an individual survives longer than some specified time t. $S(t)$ gives the probability that the random variable T (survival time) exceeds the specified time t. In other words, the survival function provides a prediction for the percentage of people expected to "survive" to a particular time.
- T is the random variable for a person's survival time.
- t represents any specific value of interest for the random variable T.

19. **List the properties of all survivor functions.**
    - Survivor functions are nonincreasing.
    - At time $t = 0$, $S(t) = S(0) = 1$. At the start of the study, the probability of surviving past $t = 0$ is one since no one has had the event yet. That is, everyone is a survivor at time $= 0$.
    - At time $= \infty$, $S(t) = S(\infty) = 0$. If the study period were increased without limit, nobody would survive.

20. **What is the hazard function?**
    The hazard function calculates the hazard (a probability) that an individual who is under observation at a time t has an event at that time. The hazard function represents the instantaneous event rate for an individual who has already survived to time t.

21. **What is the conditional failure rate?**
    The conditional failure rate is another name for the hazard function. Another way of saying this is that the conditional failure rate $h(t)$ gives the instantaneous potential for failing at time t per unit time, given survival up to time t.

22. **How is the hazard function mathematically defined?**
    The hazard function is defined by $h(t) = f(t)/S(t)$ the conditional density for T, given survival up to time t, evaluated at that time. An equivalent definition is

$$h(t) = \lim_{\delta t \to 0} \frac{P(T < t + \delta t | T = t)}{\delta t}$$

23. **Explain why the hazard function is a rate rather than a probability.**
    The numerator for this function is the conditional probability. The denominator denotes a small time interval. By division, probability per unit of time becomes a rate. The scale for this ratio ranges between 0 and infinity.

24. **How does the hazard function differ from the survivor function?**
    The survivor function gives the percentage of the subjects not having an event, whereas the hazard function gives an event rate. The hazard relates to the incident (current) event rate, whereas survival reflects the cumulative nonoccurrence.

KEY POINTS: SURVIVAL ANALYSIS

1. Survival analysis quantifies time to a single dichotomous event.

2. It handles censored data well.

3. Survival and hazard can be mathematically converted to each other.

4. Kaplan-Meier survival curves can be compared statistically and graphically.

5. Cox proportional hazards models help distinguish individual contributions of covariates on survival, provided certain assumptions are met.

25. **List the characteristics of the hazard function.**
    - It is always ≥ 0.
    - It has no upper bound because it is a rate and not a probability, as expressed in the formula.

26. **Name and graph the different types of hazard functions.**
   - Exponential survival model (Fig. 19-2.): The hazard function is constant. This is an example of h(t) for healthy persons. A person who continues to be healthy throughout the study has a constant instantaneous potential for becoming ill during the time period.
   - Increasing Weibull model (Fig. 19-3.): An example of this type of graph is cancer patients not responding to treatment, where the event of interest is death. A patient's potential for death from the disease increases as survival time increases because the prognosis worsens.
   - Decreasing Weibull model (Fig. 19-4.): This type of graph can be expected in persons recovering from surgery, where the event of interest is death. The potential for dying after surgery decreases as the time after surgery increases.
   - Lognormal survival model (Fig. 19-5): An example of this type of graph is patients who have a disease in which the potential for dying increases early in the disease and decreases later.

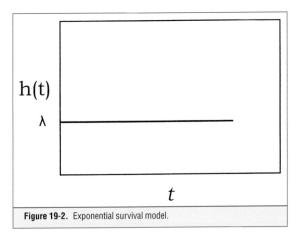

Figure 19-2. Exponential survival model.

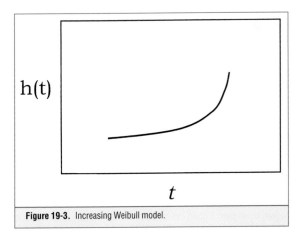

Figure 19-3. Increasing Weibull model.

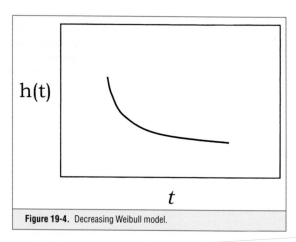

Figure 19-4. Decreasing Weibull model.

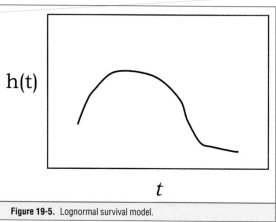

Figure 19-5. Lognormal survival model.

27. **What is the mathematic relationship between S(t) and h(t)?**

$$h(t) = \frac{-[dS(t)/dt]}{S(t)}$$

For the mathematically inclined, if the equation is rearranged and integrated, a cumulative hazard rate H(t) integrated over time t can be found to equal the natural log of S(t).

28. **What are the two basic survival procedures that enable one to determine overall single group survival, taking into account both censored and uncensored observations?**
   - Life table analysis (or actuarial)
   - Kaplan-Meier survival curve method

29. **What is a life table analysis?**
   The life table technique gives a good indication of the distribution of failures over time. It involves dividing the total period over which a group is observed into fixed intervals. For each interval, the proportion surviving at the end of the interval is calculated based on the number

known to have experienced the endpoint event during the interval and the number estimated to have been at risk as the start of the interval.

All loss and gain of subjects is assumed to occur randomly throughout the interval; therefore, the observed period is estimated as the mean value of the interval time.

Figure 19-6 shows the life table or actuarial method of survival analysis, used in the Veterans Administration Coronary Artery Bypass Surgery Cooperative Study.

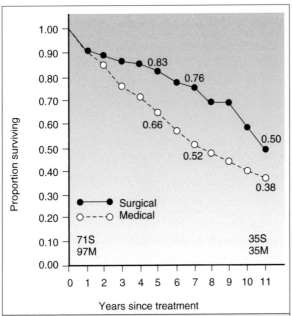

Figure 19-6. Actuary method of survival analysis, used in the Veterans Administration Coronary Artery Bypass Surgery Cooperative Study. (From Jekel JF, Katz DL, Elmore JG: Epidemiology, Biostatistics, and Preventive Medicine, 2nd ed. Philadelphia, W.B. Saunders, 2001, p 188, Fig. 11-4.)

30. What is the Kaplan-Meier product-limit estimator?
The Kaplan-Meier method allows the estimation of the survival function directly from the continuous survival or failure times. It provides for calculating the proportion surviving to each point in time that a failure or event occurs, rather than at fixed intervals, and generates the characteristic "stair-step" survival curves.

31. What is the advantage of the Kaplan-Meier product-limit over the life table method?
The advantage of the Kaplan-Meier product-limit over the life table method for analyzing survival and failure time data is that the resulting estimates do not depend on the grouping of the data into a certain number of time intervals. The Kaplan-Meier method and the life table method are identical if the intervals of the life table contain at most one observation.

32. Give an example of calculation of Kaplan-Meier survival time estimates.
You are interested in determining the time to clotting of the dialysis filter in patients starting continuous dialysis. Six patients are started on continuous dialysis in the study with the

following results: patient 1 clots at 24 hours, patient 2 dies at 10 hours, patient 3 is taken off dialysis to go to surgery within 6 hours of initiating dialysis, patient 4 clots at 42 hours, patient 5 clots after 9 hours of starting dialysis, patient 6 clots after 10 hours, patient 7 clots at 6 hours, patient 8 clots at 2 hours, patient 9 clots at 12 hours, and patient 10 clots at 5 hours. Using this example, make a table of the censored and noncensored data (Table 19-1).

The answer would look like Table 19-1.

TABLE 19-1. CENSORED AND NONCENSORED DATA

Patient Number	Censored (Yes / No)	Time to Event / Censoring
1	No	24 hours
2	Yes	10 hours
3	Yes	6 hours
4	No	42 hours
5	No	9 hours
6	No	10 hours
7	No	6 hours
8	No	2 hours
9	No	12 hours
10	No	5 hours

33. **Order the above example by event and censoring time.**
    See Table 19-2.

TABLE 19-2. ORDERING OF DATA BY EVENT AND CENSORING TIME

Time	Event	Censor	At Risk	Conditional probability of event	Cumulative probability
2	1	0	10	1/10 (0.10)	0.10
5	1	0	9	1/9 (0.11)	$0.10 + 0.11(1 - 0.10) = 0.20$
6	2	1	8	2/8 (0.25)	$0.20 + 0.25(1 - 0.9) = 0.23$
10	1	1	5	1/5 (0.20)	$0.23 + 0.20(1 - 0.23) = 0.38$
12	1	0	3	1/3 (0.33)	$0.38 + 0.33(1 - 0.38) = 0.59$
24	1	0	2	1/2 (0.5)	$0.59 + 0.50(1 - 0.59) = 0.80$
42	1	0	1	1/1 (1)	$0.80 + 1(1 - 0.8) = 1$

34. **What is the median time to clotting in the above example?**
    Using the cumulative probability column, the median time to clotting (i.e., the time when 50% of the filters are clotted) is somewhere between 10 and 12 hours because 50% falls between the cumulative probability of 38% and 59%.

35. **How is the Kaplan-Meier curve represented?**
    - The curve is graphed in step function (Fig. 19-7).
    - Time is on the x-axis.

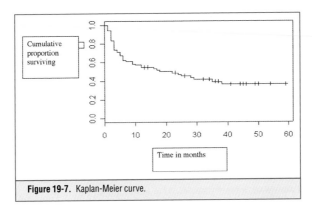

Figure 19-7. Kaplan-Meier curve.

- Cumulative probability or "survival" is on the y-axis.
- Subjects censored are represented as tick marks.
- The number of subjects "at risk" is often recorded below the x-axis.

36. **What is the limitation of the Kaplan-Meier survival curve?**
It does not account for confounding or effect modification by other covariates.

37. **When might one want to compare two different survival curves?**
When one wants to compare survival time among different groups.

38. **How are Kaplan-Meier curves from two different groups compared statistically?**
The log rank test provides overall comparison of Kaplan-Meier curves. It is a large-sample chi-square test that compares observed versus expected outcomes, where categories are defined by ordered failure times for an entire set of data. Comparisons are done at every "event" point.

39. **What are the assumptions of the log rank test?**
- The survival times are ordinal or continuous.
- The risk of an event in one group relative to the other does not change with time. This is known as the proportional hazards assumption.

40. **What are other tests used to compare survival curves?**
- The Mantel-Haenszel log rank test
- The hazard ratio

41. **What is the hazard ratio?**
The hazard ratio is the measure of effect in survival analysis that describes the exposure-outcome relationship. A hazard ratio of 1 means no effect. A hazard ratio of 5 indicates that the exposed group has 5 times the hazard of the unexposed group. A hazard ratio of 1/5 indicates that the exposed group has one fifth the hazard of the unexposed group.

42. **How do you assess relationships among several covariates and survival time?**
The Cox proportional hazards regression model is used to assess the effect of multiple covariates on survival.

WEBSITES

1. http://www.apha.org/public_health/epidemiology.htm
2. http://www.amstat.org/sections/epi/SIE_Home.htm
3. http://www.apic.org
4. http://www.biostat.ucsf.edu/epidem/epidem.html

BIBLIOGRAPHY

1. Gordis L: Epidemiology, 3rd ed. Philadelphia, W.B. Saunders, 2004.
2. Jekel JF, Katz DL, Elmore JG: Epidemiology, Biostatistics, and Preventive Medicine, 2nd ed. Philadelphia, W.B. Saunders, 2001.

APPENDIX A

TABLE A	STANDARD NORMAL–TAIL PROBABILITIES (TABLE OF z VALUES)*				
z	Upper-Tail Probability	Two-Tailed Probability	z	Upper-Tail Probability	Two-Tailed Probability
0.00	0.5000	1.0000	0.23	0.4090	0.8181
0.01	0.4960	0.9920	0.24	0.4052	0.8103
0.02	0.4920	0.9840	0.25	0.4013	0.8026
0.0251	0.49	0.98	0.2533	0.40	0.80
0.03	0.4880	0.9761	0.26	0.3974	0.7949
0.04	0.4840	0.9681	0.27	0.3936	0.7872
0.05	0.4801	0.9601	0.2793	0.39	0.78
0.0502	0.48	0.96	0.28	0.3897	0.7795
0.06	0.4761	0.9522	0.29	0.3859	0.7718
0.07	0.4721	0.9442	0.30	0.3821	0.7642
0.0753	0.47	0.94	0.3055	0.38	0.76
0.08	0.4681	0.9362	0.31	0.3783	0.7566
0.09	0.4641	0.9283	0.32	0.3745	0.7490
0.10	0.4602	0.9203	0.33	0.3707	0.7414
0.1004	0.46	0.92	0.3319	0.37	0.74
0.11	0.4562	0.9124	0.34	0.3669	0.7339
0.12	0.4522	0.9045	0.35	0.3632	0.7263
0.1257	0.45	0.9	0.3585	0.36	0.72
0.13	0.4483	0.8966	0.36	0.3594	0.7188
0.14	0.4443	0.8887	0.37	0.3557	0.7114
0.15	0.4404	0.8808	0.38	0.3520	0.7039
0.1510	0.44	0.88	0.3853	0.35	0.70
0.16	0.4364	0.8729	0.39	0.3483	0.6965
0.17	0.4325	0.8650	0.40	0.3446	0.6892
0.1764	0.43	0.86	0.41	0.3409	0.6818
0.18	0.4286	0.8571	0.4125	0.34	0.68
0.19	0.4247	0.8493	0.42	0.3372	0.6745
0.20	0.4207	0.8415	0.43	0.3336	0.6672
0.2019	0.42	0.84	0.4399	0.33	0.66
0.21	0.4168	0.8337	0.44	0.3300	0.6599
0.22	0.4129	0.8259	0.45	0.3264	0.6527
0.2275	0.41	0.82	0.46	0.3228	0.6455

Continued

TABLE A	STANDARD NORMAL–TAIL PROBABILITIES (TABLE OF z VALUES)*—CONT'D				
z	Upper-Tail Probability	Two-Tailed Probability	z	Upper-Tail Probability	Two-Tailed Probability
0.4677	0.32	0.64	0.77	0.2206	0.4413
0.47	0.3192	0.6384	0.7722	0.22	0.44
0.48	0.3156	0.6312	0.78	0.2177	0.4354
0.49	0.3121	0.6241	0.79	0.2148	0.4295
0.4959	0.31	0.62	0.80	0.2119	0.4237
0.50	0.3085	0.6171	0.8064	0.21	0.42
0.51	0.3050	0.6101	0.81	0.2090	0.4179
0.52	0.3015	0.6031	0.82	0.2061	0.4122
0.5244	0.3	0.6	0.83	0.2033	0.4065
0.53	0.2981	0.5961	0.84	0.2005	0.4009
0.54	0.2946	0.5892	0.8416	0.20	0.40
0.55	0.2912	0.5823	0.85	0.1977	0.3953
0.5534	0.29	0.58	0.86	0.1949	0.3898
0.56	0.2877	0.5755	0.87	0.1922	0.3843
0.57	0.2843	0.5687	0.8779	0.19	0.38
0.58	0.2810	0.5619	0.88	0.1894	0.3789
0.5828	0.28	0.56	0.89	0.1867	0.3735
0.59	0.2776	0.5552	0.90	0.1841	0.3681
0.60	0.2743	0.5485	0.91	0.1814	0.3628
0.61	0.2709	0.5419	0.9154	0.18	0.36
0.6128	0.27	0.54	0.92	0.1788	0.3576
0.62	0.2676	0.5353	0.93	0.1762	0.3524
0.63	0.2643	0.5287	0.94	0.1736	0.3472
0.64	0.2611	0.5222	0.95	0.1711	0.3421
0.6433	0.26	0.52	0.9542	0.17	0.34
0.65	0.2578	0.5157	0.96	0.1685	0.3371
0.66	0.2546	0.5093	0.97	0.1660	0.3320
0.67	0.2514	0.5029	0.98	0.1635	0.3271
0.6745	0.25	0.50	0.99	0.1611	0.3222
0.68	0.2483	0.4956	0.9945	0.16	0.32
0.69	0.2451	0.4902	1.00	0.1587	0.3173
0.70	0.2420	0.4839	1.01	0.1562	0.3125
0.7063	0.24	0.48	1.02	0.1539	0.3077
0.71	0.2389	0.4777	1.03	0.1515	0.3030
0.72	0.2358	0.4715	1.036	0.15	0.3
0.73	0.2327	0.4654	1.04	0.1492	0.2983
0.7388	0.23	0.46	1.05	0.1469	0.2937
0.74	0.2296	0.4593	1.06	0.1446	0.2891
0.75	0.2266	0.4533	1.07	0.1423	0.2846
0.76	0.2236	0.4473	1.08	0.1401	0.2801

TABLE A	STANDARD NORMAL–TAIL PROBABILITIES (TABLE OF z VALUES)* —CONT'D				
z	Upper-Tail Probability	Two-Tailed Probability	z	Upper-Tail Probability	Two-Tailed Probability
1.080	0.14	0.28	1.41	0.0793	0.1585
1.09	0.1379	0.2757	1.42	0.0778	0.1556
1.10	0.1357	0.2713	1.43	0.0764	0.1527
1.11	0.1335	0.2670	1.44	0.0749	0.1499
1.12	0.1314	0.2627	1.45	0.0735	0.1471
1.1264	0.13	0.26	1.46	0.0721	0.1443
1.13	0.1292	0.2585	1.47	0.0708	0.1416
1.14	0.1271	0.2543	1.476	0.07	0.14
1.15	0.1251	0.2501	1.48	0.0694	0.1389
1.16	0.1230	0.2460	1.49	0.0681	0.1362
1.17	0.1210	0.2420	1.50	0.0668	0.1336
1.175	0.12	0.24	1.51	0.0655	0.1310
1.18	0.1190	0.2380	1.52	0.0643	0.1285
1.19	0.1170	0.2340	1.53	0.0630	0.1260
1.20	0.1151	0.2301	1.54	0.0618	0.1236
1.21	0.1131	0.2263	1.55	0.0606	0.1211
1.22	0.1112	0.2225	1.555	0.06	0.12
1.227	0.11	0.22	1.56	0.0594	0.1188
1.23	0.1093	0.2187	1.57	0.0582	0.1164
1.24	0.1075	0.2150	1.58	0.0571	0.1141
1.25	0.1056	0.2113	1.59	0.0559	0.1118
1.26	0.1038	0.2077	1.60	0.0548	0.1096
1.27	0.1020	0.2041	1.61	0.0537	0.1074
1.28	0.1003	0.2005	1.62	0.0526	0.1052
1.282	0.10	0.20	1.63	0.0516	0.1031
1.29	0.0985	0.1971	1.64	0.0505	0.1010
1.30	0.0968	0.1936	1.645	0.05	0.10
1.31	0.0951	0.1902	1.65	0.0495	0.0989
1.32	0.0934	0.1868	1.66	0.0485	0.0969
1.33	0.0918	0.1835	1.67	0.0475	0.0949
1.34	0.0901	0.1802	1.68	0.0465	0.0930
1.341	0.09	0.18	1.69	0.0455	0.0910
1.35	0.0885	0.1770	1.70	0.0446	0.0891
1.36	0.0869	0.1738	1.71	0.0436	0.0873
1.37	0.0853	0.1707	1.72	0.0427	0.0854
1.38	0.0838	0.1676	1.73	0.0418	0.0836
1.39	0.0823	0.1645	1.74	0.0409	0.0819
1.40	0.0808	0.1615	1.75	0.0401	0.0801
1.405	0.08	0.16	1.751	0.04	0.08

Continued

TABLE A	STANDARD NORMAL–TAIL PROBABILITIES (TABLE OF z VALUES)* —CONT'D				
z	Upper-Tail Probability	Two-Tailed Probability	z	Upper-Tail Probability	Two-Tailed Probability
1.76	0.0392	0.0784	2.14	0.0162	0.0324
1.77	0.0384	0.0767	2.15	0.0158	0.0316
1.78	0.0375	0.0751	2.16	0.0154	0.0308
1.79	0.0367	0.0734	2.17	0.0150	0.0300
1.80	0.0359	0.0719	2.18	0.0146	0.0293
1.81	0.0352	0.0703	2.19	0.0143	0.0285
1.82	0.0344	0.0688	2.20	0.0139	0.0278
1.83	0.0336	0.0672	2.21	0.0136	0.0271
1.84	0.0329	0.0658	2.22	0.0132	0.0264
1.85	0.0322	0.0643	2.23	0.0129	0.0257
1.86	0.0314	0.0629	2.24	0.0125	0.0251
1.87	0.0307	0.0615	2.25	0.0122	0.0244
1.88	0.0301	0.0601	2.26	0.0119	0.0238
1.881	0.03	0.06	2.27	0.0116	0.0232
1.89	0.0294	0.0588	2.28	0.0113	0.0226
1.90	0.0287	0.0574	2.29	0.0110	0.0220
1.91	0.0281	0.0561	2.30	0.0107	0.0214
1.92	0.0274	0.0549	2.31	0.0104	0.0209
1.93	0.0268	0.0536	2.32	0.0102	0.0203
1.94	0.0262	0.0524	2.326	0.01	0.02
1.95	0.0256	0.0512	2.33	0.0099	0.0198
1.960	0.025	0.05	2.34	0.0096	0.0193
1.97	0.0244	0.0488	2.35	0.0094	0.0188
1.98	0.0239	0.0477	2.36	0.0091	0.0183
1.99	0.0233	0.0466	2.37	0.0089	0.0178
2.00	0.0228	0.0455	2.38	0.0087	0.0173
2.01	0.0222	0.0444	2.39	0.0084	0.0168
2.02	0.0217	0.0434	2.40	0.0082	0.0164
2.03	0.0212	0.0424	2.41	0.0080	0.0160
2.04	0.0207	0.0414	2.42	0.0078	0.0155
2.05	0.0202	0.0404	2.43	0.0075	0.0151
2.054	0.02	0.04	2.44	0.0073	0.0147
2.06	0.0197	0.0394	2.45	0.0071	0.0143
2.07	0.0192	0.0385	2.46	0.0069	0.0139
2.08	0.0188	0.0375	2.47	0.0068	0.0135
2.09	0.0183	0.0366	2.48	0.0066	0.0131
2.10	0.0179	0.0357	2.49	0.0064	0.0128
2.11	0.0174	0.0349	2.50	0.0062	0.0124
2.12	0.0170	0.0340	2.51	0.0060	0.0121
2.13	0.0166	0.0332	2.52	0.0059	0.0117

TABLE A STANDARD NORMAL-TAIL PROBABILITIES (TABLE OF z VALUES)*—CONT'D

z	Upper-Tail Probability	Two-Tailed Probability	z	Upper-Tail Probability	Two-Tailed Probability
2.53	0.0057	0.0114	3.00	0.0013	0.0027
2.54	0.0055	0.0111	3.05	0.0011	0.0023
2.55	0.0054	0.0108	3.090	0.001	0.002
2.56	0.0052	0.0105	3.10	0.0010	0.0019
2.57	0.0051	0.0102	3.15	0.0008	0.0016
2.576	0.005	0.01	3.20	0.0007	0.0014
2.58	0.0049	0.0099	3.25	0.0006	0.0012
2.59	0.0048	0.0096	3.291	0.0005	0.001
2.60	0.0047	0.0093	3.30	0.0005	0.0010
2.61	0.0045	0.0091	3.35	0.0004	0.0008
2.62	0.0044	0.0088	3.40	0.0003	0.0007
2.63	0.0043	0.0085	3.45	0.0003	0.0006
2.64	0.0041	0.0083	3.50	0.0002	0.0005
2.65	0.0040	0.0080	3.55	0.0002	0.0004
2.70	0.0035	0.0069	3.60	0.0002	0.0003
2.75	0.0030	0.0060	3.65	0.0001	0.0003
2.80	0.0026	0.0051	3.70	0.0001	0.0002
2.85	0.0022	0.0044	3.75	0.0001	0.0002
2.90	0.0019	0.0037	3.80	0.0001	0.0001
2.95	0.0016	0.0032			

Source of data: National Bureau of Standards. Applied Mathematics Series—23. US Government Printing Office, Washington, D. C., 1953. Abstracted by Shott, S. Statistics for Health Professionals. Philadelphia, W. B. Saunders Company, 1990. Used by permission.

*Instructions for use of the table to determine the *p* value that corresponds to a calculated *z* value: In the left-hand column (headed *z*), look up the value of *z* found from calculations. Look at the first column to the right (for a one-tailed *p* value) or the second column to the right (for a two-tailed *p* value) that corresponds to the value of *z* obtained. For example, a *z* value of 1.74 corresponds to a two-tailed *p* value of 0.0819.

Instructions for use of the table to determine the *z* value that corresponds to a chosen *p* value: To find the appropriate *z* value for use in confidence limits or sample size determinations, define the one-tailed or two-tailed *p* value desired, look that up in the second or third column, respectively, and determine the *z* value on the left that corresponds. For example, for a two-tailed alpha at 0.05, the corresponding *z* is 1.960; and for a one-tailed beta of 0.20, the corresponding *z* is 0.8416.

APPENDIX B

TABLE B	UPPER PERCENTAGE POINTS FOR t DISTRIBUTIONS*						
	Upper-Tail Probability						
df	0.40	0.30	0.20	0.15	0.10	0.05	0.025
1	0.325	0.727	1.376	1.963	3.078	6.314	12.706
2	0.289	0.617	1.061	1.386	1.886	2.920	4.303
3	0.277	0.584	0.978	1.250	1.638	2.353	3.182
4	0.271	0.569	0.941	1.190	1.533	2.132	2.776
5	0.267	0.559	0.920	1.156	1.476	2.015	2.571
6	0.265	0.553	0.906	1.134	1.440	1.943	2.447
7	0.263	0.549	0.896	1.119	1.415	1.895	2.365
8	0.262	0.546	0.889	1.108	1.397	1.860	2.306
9	0.261	0.543	0.883	1.100	1.383	1.833	2.262
10	0.260	0.542	0.879	1.093	1.372	1.812	2.228
11	0.260	0.540	0.876	1.088	1.363	1.796	2.201
12	0.259	0.539	0.873	1.083	1.356	1.782	2.179
13	0.259	0.537	0.870	1.079	1.350	1.771	2.160
14	0.258	0.537	0.868	1.076	1.345	1.761	2.145
15	0.258	0.536	0.866	1.074	1.341	1.753	2.131
16	0.258	0.535	0.865	1.071	1.337	1.746	2.120
17	0.257	0.534	0.863	1.069	1.333	1.740	2.110
18	0.257	0.534	0.862	1.067	1.330	1.734	2.101
19	0.257	0.533	0.861	1.066	1.328	1.729	2.093
20	0.257	0.533	0.860	1.064	1.325	1.725	2.086
21	0.257	0.532	0.859	1.063	1.323	1.721	2.080
22	0.256	0.532	0.858	1.061	1.321	1.717	2.074
23	0.256	0.532	0.858	1.060	1.319	1.714	2.069
24	0.256	0.531	0.857	1.059	1.318	1.711	2.064
25	0.256	0.531	0.856	1.058	1.316	1.708	2.060
26	0.256	0.531	0.856	1.058	1.315	1.706	2.056
27	0.256	0.531	0.855	1.057	1.314	1.703	2.052
28	0.256	0.530	0.855	1.056	1.313	1.701	2.048
29	0.256	0.530	0.854	1.055	1.311	1.699	2.045
30	0.256	0.530	0.854	1.055	1.310	1.697	2.042
40	0.255	0.529	0.851	1.050	1.303	1.684	2.021
60	0.254	0.527	0.848	1.045	1.296	1.671	2.000
120	0.254	0.526	0.845	1.041	1.289	1.658	1.980
∞	0.253	0.524	0.842	1.036	1.282	1.645	1.960

df	Upper-Tail Probability						
	0.02	0.015	0.01	0.0075	0.005	0.0025	0.0005
1	15.895	21.205	31.821	42.434	63.657	127.322	636.590
2	4.849	5.643	6.965	8.073	9.925	14.089	31.598
3	3.482	3.896	4.541	5.047	5.841	7.453	12.924
4	2.999	3.298	3.747	4.088	4.604	5.598	8.610
5	2.757	3.003	3.365	3.634	4.032	4.773	6.869
6	2.612	2.829	3.143	3.372	3.707	4.317	5.959
7	2.517	2.715	2.998	3.203	3.499	4.029	5.408
8	2.449	2.634	2.896	3.085	3.355	3.833	5.041
9	2.398	2.574	2.821	2.998	3.250	3.690	4.781
10	2.359	2.527	2.764	2.932	3.169	3.581	4.587
11	2.328	2.491	2.718	2.879	3.106	3.497	4.437
12	2.303	2.461	2.681	2.836	3.055	3.428	4.318
13	2.282	2.436	2.650	2.801	3.012	3.372	4.221
14	2.264	2.415	2.624	2.771	2.977	3.326	4.140
15	2.249	2.397	2.602	2.746	2.947	3.286	4.073
16	2.235	2.382	2.583	2.724	2.921	3.252	4.015
17	2.224	2.368	2.567	2.706	2.898	3.222	3.965
18	2.214	2.356	2.552	2.689	2.878	3.197	3.922
19	2.205	2.346	2.539	2.674	2.861	3.174	3.883
20	2.197	2.336	2.528	2.661	2.845	3.153	3.849
21	2.189	2.328	2.518	2.649	2.831	3.135	3.819
22	2.183	2.320	2.508	2.639	2.819	3.119	3.792
23	2.177	2.313	2.500	2.629	2.807	3.104	3.768
24	2.172	2.307	2.492	2.620	2.797	3.091	3.745
25	2.167	2.301	2.485	2.612	2.787	3.078	3.725
26	2.162	2.296	2.479	2.605	2.779	3.067	3.707
27	2.158	2.291	2.473	2.598	2.771	3.057	3.690
28	2.154	2.286	2.467	2.592	2.763	3.047	3.674
29	2.150	2.282	2.462	2.586	2.756	3.038	3.659
30	2.147	2.278	2.457	2.581	2.750	3.030	3.646
40	2.123	2.250	2.423	2.542	2.704	2.971	3.551
60	2.099	2.223	2.390	2.504	2.660	2.915	3.460
120	2.076	2.196	2.358	2.468	2.617	2.860	3.373
∞	2.054	2.170	2.326	2.432	2.576	2.807	3.291

Source: Shott, S. Statistics for Health Professionals. Philadelphia, W. B. Saunders, 1990. Used by permission.

*Instructions for use of the table: To determine the p value that corresponds to a calculated t value, first find the line that corresponds to the column of degrees of freedom *(df)* on the left. Then in the center of the table find the value that most closely corresponds to the value of t found from calculations. **(1) For a one-tailed t-test:** Look at the top row to find the corresponding probability. For example, a t value of 2.147 on 30 *df* corresponds to a p value of 0.02. If the observed value of t falls between values given, state the two p values between which the results of the t-test fall. For example, if a t of 2.160 is found on 30 *df*, the probability is expressed as follows: $0.015 < p < 0.02$. **(2) For a two-tailed t-test:** The procedure is the same as for a one-tailed test, except that the p value obtained must then be *doubled* to include the other tail probability. For example, if a two-tailed t-test gives a t value of 2.147 on 30 *df*, the p value of that column (0.02) must be doubled to give the correct p value of 0.04.

APPENDIX C

See pages 244–247 for Table C.

TABLE C UPPER PERCENTAGE POINTS FOR CHI-SQUARE DISTRIBUTIONS*

df	Probability								
	0.9995	0.995	0.99	0.975	0.95	0.90	0.80	0.70	0.60
1	0.000000393	0.0000393	0.000157	0.000982	0.00393	0.0158	0.0642	0.148	0.275
2	0.00100	0.0100	0.0201	0.0506	0.103	0.211	0.446	0.713	1.022
3	0.0153	0.0717	0.115	0.216	0.352	0.584	1.005	1.424	1.869
4	0.0639	0.207	0.297	0.484	0.711	1.064	1.649	2.195	2.753
5	0.158	0.412	0.554	0.831	1.145	1.610	2.343	3.000	3.655
6	0.299	0.676	0.872	1.237	1.635	2.204	3.070	3.828	4.570
7	0.485	0.989	1.239	1.690	2.167	2.833	3.822	4.671	5.493
8	0.710	1.344	1.646	2.180	2.733	3.490	4.594	5.527	6.423
9	0.972	1.735	2.088	2.700	3.325	4.168	5.380	6.393	7.357
10	1.265	2.156	2.558	3.247	3.940	4.865	6.179	7.267	8.295
11	1.587	2.603	3.053	3.816	4.575	5.578	6.989	8.148	9.237
12	1.934	3.074	3.571	4.404	5.226	6.304	7.807	9.034	10.182
13	2.305	3.565	4.107	5.009	5.892	7.042	8.634	9.926	11.129
14	2.697	4.075	4.660	5.629	6.571	7.790	9.467	10.821	12.078
15	3.108	4.601	5.229	6.262	7.261	8.547	10.307	11.721	13.030
16	3.536	5.142	5.812	6.908	7.962	9.312	11.152	12.624	13.983
17	3.980	5.697	6.408	7.564	8.672	10.085	12.002	13.531	14.937
18	4.439	6.265	7.015	8.231	9.390	10.865	12.857	14.440	15.893
19	4.912	6.844	7.633	8.907	10.117	11.651	13.716	15.352	16.850
20	5.398	7.434	8.260	9.591	10.851	12.443	14.578	16.266	17.809
21	5.896	8.034	8.897	10.283	11.591	13.240	15.445	17.182	18.768
22	6.404	8.643	9.542	10.982	12.338	14.041	16.314	18.101	19.729

TABLE C	UPPER PERCENTAGE POINTS FOR CHI-SQUARE DISTRIBUTIONS* —CONT'D								
					Probability				
df	0.9995	0.995	0.99	0.975	0.95	0.90	0.80	0.70	0.60
23	6.924	9.260	10.196	11.689	13.091	14.848	17.187	19.021	20.690
24	7.453	9.886	10.856	12.401	13.848	15.659	18.062	19.943	21.652
25	7.991	10.520	11.524	13.120	14.611	16.473	18.940	20.867	22.616
26	8.538	11.160	12.198	13.844	15.379	17.292	19.820	21.792	23.579
27	9.093	11.808	12.879	14.573	16.151	18.114	20.703	22.719	24.544
28	9.656	12.461	13.565	15.308	16.928	18.939	21.588	23.647	25.509
29	10.227	13.121	14.256	16.047	17.708	19.768	22.475	24.577	26.475
30	10.804	13.787	14.953	16.791	18.493	20.599	23.364	25.508	27.442
35	13.787	17.192	18.509	20.569	22.465	24.797	27.836	30.178	32.282
40	16.906	20.707	22.164	24.433	26.509	29.051	32.345	34.872	37.134
45	20.137	24.311	25.901	28.366	30.612	33.350	36.884	39.585	41.995
50	23.461	27.991	29.707	32.357	34.764	37.689	41.449	44.313	46.864
60	30.340	35.534	37.485	40.482	43.188	46.459	50.641	53.809	56.620
70	37.467	43.275	45.442	48.758	51.739	55.329	59.898	63.346	66.396
80	44.791	51.172	53.540	57.153	60.391	64.278	69.207	72.915	76.188
90	52.276	59.196	61.754	65.647	69.126	73.291	78.558	82.511	85.993
100	59.896	67.328	70.065	74.222	77.929	82.358	87.945	92.129	95.808
120	75.467	83.852	86.923	91.573	95.705	100.624	106.806	111.419	115.465
140	91.391	100.655	104.034	109.137	113.659	119.029	125.758	130.766	135.149
160	107.597	117.679	121.346	126.870	131.756	137.546	144.783	150.158	154.856
180	124.033	134.884	138.820	144.741	149.969	156.153	163.868	169.588	174.580
200	140.660	152.241	156.432	162.728	168.279	174.835	183.003	189.049	194.319

df	Probability									
	0.50	0.40	0.30	0.20	0.10	0.05	0.025	0.01	0.005	0.005
1	0.455	0.708	1.074	1.642	2.706	3.841	5.024	6.635	7.879	12.116
2	1.386	1.833	2.408	3.219	4.605	5.991	7.378	9.210	10.597	15.202
3	2.366	2.946	3.665	4.642	6.251	7.815	9.348	11.345	12.838	17.730
4	3.357	4.045	4.878	5.989	7.779	9.488	11.143	13.277	14.860	19.997
5	4.351	5.132	6.064	7.289	9.236	11.070	12.833	15.086	16.750	22.105
6	5.348	6.211	7.231	8.558	10.645	12.592	14.449	16.812	18.548	24.103
7	6.346	7.283	8.383	9.803	12.017	14.067	16.013	18.475	20.278	26.018
8	7.344	8.351	9.524	11.030	13.362	15.507	17.535	20.090	21.955	27.868
9	8.343	9.414	10.656	12.242	14.684	16.919	19.023	21.666	23.589	29.666
10	9.342	10.473	11.781	13.442	15.987	18.307	20.483	23.209	25.188	31.420
11	10.341	11.530	12.899	14.631	17.275	19.675	21.920	24.725	26.757	33.137
12	11.340	12.584	14.011	15.812	18.549	21.026	23.337	26.217	28.300	34.821
13	12.340	13.636	15.119	16.985	19.812	22.362	24.736	27.688	29.819	36.478
14	13.339	14.685	16.222	18.151	21.064	23.685	26.119	29.141	31.319	38.109
15	14.339	15.733	17.322	19.311	22.307	24.996	27.488	30.578	32.801	39.719
16	15.338	16.780	18.418	20.465	23.542	26.296	28.845	32.000	34.267	41.308
17	16.338	17.824	19.511	21.615	24.769	27.587	30.191	33.409	35.718	42.879
18	17.338	18.868	20.601	22.760	25.989	28.869	31.526	34.805	37.156	44.434
19	18.338	19.910	21.689	23.900	27.204	30.144	32.852	36.191	38.582	45.973
20	19.337	20.951	22.775	25.038	28.412	31.410	34.170	37.566	39.997	47.498
21	20.337	21.991	23.858	26.171	29.615	32.671	35.479	38.932	41.401	49.011
22	21.337	23.031	24.939	27.301	30.813	33.924	36.781	40.289	42.796	50.511
23	22.337	24.069	26.018	28.429	32.007	35.172	38.076	41.638	44.181	52.000
24	23.337	25.106	27.096	29.553	33.196	36.415	39.364	42.980	45.559	53.479
25	24.337	26.143	28.172	30.675	34.382	37.652	40.646	44.314	46.928	54.947
26	25.336	27.179	29.246	31.795	35.563	38.885	41.923	45.642	48.290	56.407

TABLE C   UPPER PERCENTAGE POINTS FOR CHI-SQUARE DISTRIBUTIONS —CONT'D

df	Probability									
	0.9995	0.995	0.99	0.975	0.95	0.90	0.80	0.70	0.60	0.50
27	57.858	49.645	46.963	43.195	40.113	36.741	32.912	30.319	28.214	26.336
28	59.300	50.993	48.278	44.461	41.337	37.916	34.027	31.391	29.249	27.336
29	60.735	52.336	49.588	45.722	42.557	39.087	35.139	32.461	30.283	28.336
30	62.162	53.672	50.892	46.979	43.773	40.256	36.250	33.530	31.316	29.336
35	69.199	60.275	57.342	53.203	49.802	46.059	41.778	38.859	36.475	34.336
40	76.095	66.766	63.691	59.342	55.758	51.805	47.269	44.165	41.622	39.335
45	82.876	73.166	69.957	65.410	61.656	57.505	52.729	49.452	46.761	44.335
50	89.561	79.490	76.154	71.420	67.505	63.167	58.164	54.723	51.892	49.335
60	102.695	91.952	88.379	83.298	79.082	74.397	68.972	65.227	62.135	59.335
70	115.578	104.215	100.425	95.023	90.531	85.527	79.715	75.689	72.358	69.334
80	128.261	116.321	112.329	106.629	101.879	96.578	90.405	86.120	82.566	79.334
90	140.782	128.299	124.116	118.136	113.145	107.565	101.054	96.524	92.761	89.334
100	153.167	140.169	135.807	129.561	124.342	118.498	111.667	106.906	102.946	99.334
120	177.603	163.648	158.950	152.211	146.567	140.233	132.806	127.616	123.289	119.334
140	201.683	186.847	181.840	174.648	168.613	161.827	153.854	148.269	143.604	139.334
160	225.481	209.824	204.530	196.915	190.516	183.311	174.828	168.876	163.898	159.334
180	249.048	232.620	227.056	219.044	212.304	204.704	195.743	189.446	184.173	179.334
200	272.423	255.264	249.445	241.058	233.994	226.021	216.609	209.985	204.434	199.334

Source of data: Copyright 1982, Novartis. Reprinted with permission from the Geigy Scientific Tables, 8th ed., edited by Lentner, C. All rights reserved. Abstracted by Shott, S. Statistics for Health Professionals, Philadelphia. W. B. Saunders Company, 1990.

*Instructions for use of the table: Determine the degrees of freedom (df) appropriate to the chi-square test just calculated, and go to the line that most closely corresponds, using the left-hand column (headed df). On that line, move to the right in the body of the table and find the chi-square value that corresponds to what was calculated. The corresponding p value is found at the top of that column. For example, on 6 df, a calculated chi-square of 12.592 corresponds to a p value of 0.05. If the calculated chi-square value falls between two columns in the table, state the two p values between which the results of the chi-square test fall. For example, on 6 df, the probability of a chi-square of 13.500 is expressed as follows: 0.025 < p < 0.05.

INDEX

Page numbers in **boldface type** indicate complete chapters.